Clinical Learning and Teaching Innovations in Nursing

Innovation and Change in Professional Education

VOLUME 10

SCOPE OF THE SERIES

The primary aim of this book series is to provide a platform for exchanging experiences and knowledge about educational innovation and change in professional education and post-secondary education (engineering, law, medicine, management, health sciences, etc.). The series provides an opportunity to publish reviews, issues of general significance to theory development and research in professional education, and critical analysis of professional practice to the enhancement of educational innovation in the professions.

The series promotes publications that deal with pedagogical issues that arise in the context of innovation and change of professional education. It publishes work from leading practitioners in the field, and cutting edge researchers. Each volume is dedicated to a specific theme in professional education, providing a convenient resource of publications dedicated to further development of professional education.

For further volumes:
http://www.springer.com/series/6087

Kay Edgecombe • Margaret Bowden
Editors

Clinical Learning and Teaching Innovations in Nursing

Dedicated Education Units Building a Better Future

Springer

Editors
Kay Edgecombe
School of Nursing and Midwifery
Flinders University
Adelaide, South Australia
Australia

Margaret Bowden
School of Nursing and Midwifery
Flinders University
Adelaide, South Australia
Australia

ISBN 978-94-007-7231-1 ISBN 978-94-007-7232-8 (eBook)
DOI 10.1007/978-94-007-7232-8
Springer Dordrecht Heidelberg New York London

Printed on acid-free paper

Springer is part of Springer Science+Business Media (www.springer.com)

Preface

The Dedicated Education Unit (DEU) is an example of the increasing adoption of work-integrated learning concepts and practices as the way forward in preparing higher education students for real-world nursing. It was born from the complexities of providing more students with more quality time in fewer clinical practice settings with fewer resources whilst ensuring a greater number and range of hands-on nursing experiences, greater numbers of work ready graduate Registered Nurses (RNs) and reduced costs. Rather than being a proscriptive model, the DEU was conceptualised and has continued to develop as a flexible clinical learning and teaching strategy informed by the philosophies and principles of adult learning, transformational learning, work-integrated learning and learning in communities of practice.

Practitioners—nurses, educators, administrators and students—who are passionate about sharing the philosophy of the DEU in nursing have collaborated to write this book. Their primary aim is to provide a resource for all those involved with student nurse education—nurse educators in the clinical setting, nurses, students, academics, ward/unit managers in hospitals, community health-care provider managers, placement coordinators, student and nurse administrators, academic and health-care policy makers and regulators. To this end, they present practice examples and personal experiences from DEUs at Flinders University and Canberra University in Australia; the University of Portland, Oregon, in the USA; New Zealand's Christchurch Polytechnic Institute of Technology and Canterbury District Health Board collaboration (CPIT/CDHB) as well as the Counties Manukau District Health Board (CMDHB)[1] and Manukau Institute of Technology (MIT) collaboration; and the University of Borås, Sweden. The examples demonstrate how different DEUs are set up, managed and constantly adapted specifically to meet the needs of varied nurse education programmes and clinical learning contexts.

[1]Since this book was written, the Counties Manukau District Health Board (CMDHB) has changed its name to Counties Manukau Health.

The authors blend pedagogy with lived experiences of DEUs as they trace the development and implementation of this clinical education partnership between tertiary education and health-care institutions. They emphasise the importance of collaboration, cooperation, collegiality, constructive criticism and shared offering of solutions to problems based on what members of the DEU 'community' know or do not know.

In all cases, the DEU philosophy has been used to build clinical environments that recognise the value of nurses, academics and peers as collaborative teachers and learners and to utilise these inbuilt resources to provide repetition in learning and develop a common sense of belonging in the 'unit'. This enables students to explore learning opportunities in the knowledge that there are people who will ensure they do not make intractable errors and who will guide and support them to achieve the competence and confidence required of graduating RNs. There have been some anecdotal reports that staff/faculty development opportunities (capacity building) in DEUs improve ward culture and reduce injuries.

Comparisons between the principles and characteristics of the DEU and other clinical nursing education 'models' highlight the DEU's unique aspects. Illustrations depicting key elements of the DEU learning and teaching environment and outlining role descriptions and responsibilities for key personnel in different DEUs provide a comprehensive guide to laying the foundations of a DEU.

The book culminates in a 'how to' chapter in the form of a sample of a DEU in practice. However, this is not a recipe book on how to do 'the' DEU. Instead, it demonstrates how flexible development and implementation of DEUs can meet the needs of different clinical learning contexts, adapting to inevitable contextual changes. The DEU concept, its philosophical and pedagogical bases and its processes may be useful for all disciplines with a work-integrated learning component. Further research and development of DEUs is intended with the aim of implementing inter-professional DEUs in clinical settings and beyond.

Kay Edgecombe and Margaret Bowden (editors)

Acknowledgements

We value the vision, passion and dedication of all who have worked to ensure the Dedicated Education Unit (DEU) concept has become a practice reality.

Kay Edgecombe and **Margaret Bowden** wish to acknowledge the hard work of all those who have contributed to this book.

Kay Edgecombe also wishes to acknowledge all the Flinders University School of Nursing and Midwifery colleagues, industry partners, nursing staff, administrators and students in Adelaide, South Australia, who supported the development, piloting and subsequent implementation of Dedicated Education Units (DEUs). Taking the risk of trying something new is always a daunting prospect, but your dedication to seeking better alternatives to nursing practice learning and teaching has led to the national and international uptake of DEUs.

The Canberra, Australia, Dedicated Education Units (DEUs) would like to acknowledge all of the nursing students, industry partners and nursing and allied health staff in Canberra who have supported the DEUs and who were willing to suspend assumptions to engage with a different way of supporting learning and practice in the clinical context.

The Canterbury Dedicated Education Unit Working Group (New Zealand) wishes to acknowledge:

Members of the original DEU Governance Group: Mary Gordon, Canterbury District Health Board (CDHB) Executive Director of Nursing; Cathy Andrew, Christchurch Institute of Technology (CPIT), Head of School, Health and Humanities; Sue Hayward, Director of Nursing Christchurch Hospital; and Sam Powell, Nurse Manager Professional Development Unit, Christchurch Hospital.

Subsequent and ongoing Governance Group members: Al McDougal, Nursing Director Surgical, Christchurch Hospital; Diana Gunn, Director of Nursing, Burwood Hospital; and Heather Byrne, Nursing Manager, Professional Development Unit, Christchurch Hospital.

Directors of Nursing, Nurse Consultants and Charge Nurse Managers of the Dedicated Education Unit practice areas in the Canterbury Health System; initial

Dedicated Education Unit (DEU) Project and Governance Group members including Michelle Casey, Janine Hale, Isabel Jamieson and Deb Sims; subsequent and current DEU Working and Governance Group members including Teresa Kilkenny, Rose Whittle, Debbie Cook and Raylene Shaw; administration staff at the Professional Development Unit, Christchurch Hospital; Sue Imrie, Personal Assistant, Executive Director of Nursing and Executive Director of Māori and Pacific Health Canterbury District Health Board, who assisted us to write the Governance Group minutes and distribute them before monthly meetings; the Medical Illustrations Department, Christchurch Hospital, who assisted us with brochure printing, often at the last minute; Claire Freeman, Graphic Designer, Allan Bean Centre, who assisted us with logo development, colours and DEU brochure development; students who have had their clinical experience in DEU practice areas and provided evaluations; Academic Liaison Nurses (ALN) and Clinical Liaison Nurses (CLN) of the pilot project who provided evaluations; staff working in the CPIT School of Nursing; staff working in the Canterbury Health System; and Nurse Maude Association, the first community provider to establish a DEU within the Canterbury Health System.

The Dedicated Education Unit (DEU) model is built on the partnership of individuals and agencies for the mutual goal of educating nurses and providing quality care to clients. **Carol Craig** and **Susan Moscato** wish to acknowledge the faculty, staff nurses, administrators and students at Providence St. Vincent Medical Center, Providence Portland Medical Center, Portland VA Medical Center and the University of Portland who have combined their time, talents and resources to make the DEU innovation a success. We acknowledge the Schools of Nursing from around the country who have consulted with our DEU team and replicated this innovation with their clinical partners. We also wish to thank Kay Edgecombe for her vision and passion that is changing nursing education.

Margaretha Ekebergh wishes to acknowledge Maud Nilsson, RN, Lecturer in clinical nursing; Elisabeth Lindberg, RN, Lecturer in clinical nursing; Kerstin Dagborn, RN, Lecturer in clinical nursing; Birgitta Sjöberg, RN, Tutor in clinical praxis; Teja Fredenlund, Tutor in clinical praxis; Eva-Britt Wustenhagen, RN, Tutor in clinical praxis; Marianne Segenstedt, RN, Developing Manager in Health care; and Ingrid Rosengren, Head of Clinical Studies for supporting the Dedicated Education Unit (DEU) at Borås University, Sweden.

Beverley McClelland, Nurse Leader, Nursing Professional Development Unit (NPDU) at Counties Manukau District Health Board (CMDHB, now called *Counties Manukau Health*), New Zealand, wishes to give special thanks to Denise Kivell who has offered support and leadership to all during the Manukau Institute of Technology (MIT)/(CMDHB) Dedicated Education Unit (DEU) action research project and to further developing the DEU concept throughout CMDHB. We acknowledge Rose Whittle's hard work and expertise in being the project's Independent Evaluator in 2009. Rose is Clinical Manager for the School of Nursing at Christchurch Polytechnic Institute of Technology (CPIT), New Zealand.

All contributors wish to acknowledge the invaluable input of reviewers, including:

JoAnn Mulready-Shick, EdD, RN, CNE, ANEF
College of Nursing and Health Sciences
University of Massachusetts Boston
Boston, MA 02125, USA
Principal Investigator, Project PDQ, Partnering for DEU Development and Quality
Evaluating Innovations in Nursing Education program
Robert Wood Johnson Foundation
New Brunswick, NJ 08901, USA

Mulready-Shick, J., Kafel, K., Banister, G., & Mylott, L. (2009). Enhancing quality and safety competency development at the unit level: An initial evaluation of student learning and clinical teaching on dedicated education units. *Journal of Nursing Education, 48*(12), 716–719.

Glazer, G., Erickson, J. I., Mylott, L., Mulready-Shick, J., & Banister, G. (2011). Partnering and leadership core requirements for developing a Dedicated Education Unit. *Journal of Nursing Administration, 41*(10), 401–406.

Dr Susan Bridges
Dental Education & e-Learning
Faculty of Dentistry
The University of Hong Kong

Bridges, S., McGrath, C., & Whitehill, T. L. (Eds.). (2012). *Problem-based learning in clinical education: The next generation.* Dordrecht: Springer.

Beverly W. Henry, Ph.D., RD
Associate Professor, Nutrition and Dietetics
School of Family, Consumer, and Nutrition Sciences
College of Health and Human Sciences
Northern Illinois University
DeKalb, IL 60115, USA

Henry, B. W., Rooney, D. M., Eller, S., McCarthy, D. M., Seivert, N. P., Nannicelli, A. P., & Vozenilek, J. A. (2013). What patients observe about teamwork in the emergency department: Development of the PIVOT questionnaire. *Journal of Participatory Medicine, 5*, e4.

Henry, B. W., & Malu, K. M. (2011). Coaching, mentoring and supervision for workplace learning, Chapter 4. In: J. P. Hafler (Ed.), *Extraordinary learning in the workplace* (pp. 63–85). New York: Springer.

Henry, B. W., Duellman, M. C., & Smith, T. J. (2009). Nutrition-based standardized patient sessions increase counseling awareness and confidence among dietetic interns. *Topics in Clinical Nutrition, 24*(1), 25–34.

Contents

About the Authors

Chapters 1, 2, 9, 11 and 12

Kay Edgecombe, RN, DipT SACAE, BNg SACAE, MNg Flin, is a Nursing Lecturer in the School of Nursing and Midwifery, Flinders University, Adelaide, Australia. Kay has been teaching and researching nursing at Flinders University since 1987. She was instrumental in developing the concept of Dedicated Education Units (DEUs) in nursing and implementing the original DEUs in South Australia. She has been the Principal Academic (PA) at three DEUs in different hospitals in Adelaide, South Australia. Her Master's research evaluated student perceptions of the clinical learning environment in DEUs and other placement models. In 2008, Kay was awarded an Australian Learning and Teaching Council (ALTC) citation acknowledging her role in conceiving and developing DEUs. Kay is a member of the Australian Nurse Teachers' Society, South Australia.

Chapters 3 and 5

Associate Professor **Laurie Grealish**, DipNg (Alberta), CertOncNg (NSW), Grad DipNG (Armidale CAE), MNg (Canberra), Ph.D. (Canberra), is a Clinical Director and Deputy Head of Nursing and Midwifery at the University of Canberra, ACT, Australia. She has 20 years' experience as an academic, with publications in the areas of work-integrated learning, cancer nursing and palliative care. Laurie has worked in the health, government and university sectors and is recognised as a leader in the area of learning in the workplace locally, nationally and internationally. Laurie's research expertise is in the area of professional competence and workplace learning, specifically learning that occurs in the Dedicated Education Unit. Through this work, she has become acutely aware of the issues related to intercultural competence in health-care settings. She was lead on the development of the Dedicated Education Unit (DEU) model at the University of Canberra in 2003.

Kasia Bail, BNurse (Hons), GradCert HighEd, Ph.D. Candidate, Assistant Professor of Nursing, University of Canberra, has worked between clinical nursing, research and teaching in Canberra since 2001. Kasia has a passion for identifying and researching the structures which impede or enable nursing care. Her Ph.D. is looking at links between patient outcomes and nursing care. Kasia has experience in acute management of chronic illness, including palliative care, cancer and emergency nursing, as well as nursing research, education and policy. Her research interests include nurse-sensitive outcomes, dementia and delirium care, prognosis and interdisciplinary communication, nursing policy, aged care nurse practitioners and clinical models for undergraduate nurse development. **(Also Ch. 10)**

Jo Gibson, RN, BN, MAdvNsgPrac (Canberra), is an Accreditation Manager at the Australian Nursing and Midwifery Accreditation Council. Jo was formerly a Lecturer at the University of Canberra and was actively involved in coordinating both the Bachelor of Nursing programme and the professional practice experience aspects of the programme. In both of these roles, Jo was a strong advocate of the DEU model. Jo has practised clinically in varied specialties in various clinical contexts around Australia. Jo received a Churchill Fellowship in 2003 for travel to the Harvard Medical School to study a course in Palliative Care Practice and Education. Jo has a strong research interest in leadership in nursing and health care and is strongly committed to patient safety. Jo is engaged in the regulation of nursing education in Australia with a personal professional aim to work collaboratively with education providers and professional peers to enable excellence in practice through education and knowledge.

Chapters 4, 10 and 11

Dr **Judith (Judy) Gonda**, RN, RM, BApp Sci, (Phillip Institute), MN (Flinders Univ), Ph.D. (University of Queensland), is a Senior Lecturer and Assistant Head of School, Nursing, Midwifery and Paramedicine at the Australian Catholic University, Queensland, Australia. Her primary focus is teaching Master of Nursing to students. Since 1989, Judy has been teaching undergraduate and postgraduate students in tertiary education throughout Australia and the USA. In the 1990s and early 2000s, at Flinders University, South Australia, Judy was instrumental in piloting, implementing and evaluating the first Dedicated Education Units (DEUs) in a partnership between Flinders University School of Nursing and the Flinders Medical Centre. She was also involved in a collaborative programme between the Flinders University Schools of Social Work and Nursing and Midwifery to develop a workplace curriculum for nursing and social work students in mental health settings. Two of Judy's main research interests are teaching and learning in nursing and clinical education.

Chapter 5

Donna Hodgson is a credentialed MHN who has a long history of educating and mentoring undergraduate and postgraduate nurses in the field of mental health. Donna is passionate about professional development activities, and ensuring a connection exists between evidence-based theory and the practice of mental health nursing. Since commencing work in the field of mental health in 1991 with the ACT Health Directorate, Donna has worked in a variety of roles including establishing the first Nursing Clozapine coordination role under the first National Mental Health Plan, as the CNC in the acute adult inpatient unit and as a community manager. Donna has worked as the Coordinator of Mental Health Nursing Education Programmes for the past 12 years. She has additionally spent 1 year as an academic teaching Mental Health units at the University of Canberra and maintains an adjunct position there which involves teaching and assessment of students.

Alan Merritt, RN, BN, MHSc (education), is a Registered Nurse with a wide range of experience in varied nursing and health-care contexts and a particular interest in nursing in the community. Alan is a past Lecturer of the University of Canberra where he facilitated the clinical experience in a multisite, multi-programme Dedicated Education Unit (DEU) in community nursing. Alan is currently in a role that involves close collaboration with national education providers to facilitate the development and accreditation of nursing curricula. Alan's research interests are in the facilitation of learning in nursing, community nursing and the ways nurses see themselves and are seen by others. His current scholarship involves exploration of professional artistry in community nursing practice utilising methodologies that include the use of rich media to uncover the authentic work context.

Dr **Jan Taylor**, RN, RM, BAppSc (Nurs Sc), MNurs, GradCert HigherEd, Ph.D., is an Associate Professor at the University of Canberra, ACT, Australia. Jan has a passion for education and has worked in educational settings for almost two decades teaching undergraduate and postgraduate nursing and midwifery students. Her specialist teaching areas include research methods, ethics and women's health. Jan is a strong advocate for women's choices in child birthing and has been active in community health forums. Her Ph.D. research focused on the impact of fatigue on new mothers.

Chapter 6

Dr **Carol Craig**, BNSc, MSc (University of Alaska), Ph.D. (Colorado Health Sciences Center), FNP certificate (University of Wisconsin Oshkosh), is currently a Professor and Associate Dean for Undergraduate Programmes at the University of Portland, Oregon, USA. This role includes oversight of the Dedicated Education Unit programme. Carol is a master teacher with experience in a number of universities. She has expertise in curriculum development, particularly in innovation in clinical education, and has a passionate interest in Dedicated Education Units.

Dr **Susan Randles Moscato**, RN, EdD, BNSc, MNg (California), Ph.D. (Portland), was an Associate Dean for Graduate Programmes and Professor, University of Portland (UP) School of Nursing, at the time of her contributions to this book. Susan joined the faculty at UP in 1977 as an adjunct Clinical Instructor and has served in a variety of teaching and administrative roles. Susan, with UP clinical partners, was instrumental in developing the Dedicated Education Unit (DEU) concept in North America and launching the first DEUs. The Institute of Medicine of the National Academies (IOM), USA, has included her work with DEUs in 'The future of Nursing: Leading change, advancing health', 2010. The implementation and evaluation of the DEU as an innovative model of clinical education is described in Moscato, S., Miller, J., Logsdon, K., Weinberg, S., & Chorpenning, L. (2007). Dedicated Education Unit: An innovative clinical partner education model. *Nursing Outlook, 55*(1), 31–37. Recognition Program. **(Also Ch. 10)**

Chapter 7

Michelle Casey, RN, MHSc (Nsg), PG cert (Continence), is a Canterbury District Health Board (CDHB) Nurse Educator for the Christchurch Polytechnic Institute of Technology (CPIT)/CDHB Dedicated Education Unit. She is a member of the CPIT/CDHB Dedicated Education Unit Working Group and Governance Group and a Coresearcher for the Dedicated Education Unit pilot project (2006–2008). Michelle has a background in surgical, oncology and general medical nursing. She is passionate about nursing, has a special interest in Gerontology and Continence and has completed her Certificate in Continence Management (2000) and Master of Health Science (Nursing, 2004).

Deborah Sims, RN, MA (Nurs), Adv.DipN (CP), Cert. Clin Tchg, Cert. Adult Tchg, is a member of the College of Nurses, Aotearoa, who is currently employed by the Christchurch Polytechnic Institute of Technology (CPIT) School of Nursing as a Senior Nursing Lecturer and is a member of the CPIT and Canterbury District Health Board (CDHB) Dedicated Education Unit Working Group and Governance Group. Deborah has a background in medical and surgical nursing, nursing management and human resources and has an interest in clinical teaching and learning. Her Master's MA (Applied) Nursing (2000–2004) research explored 'The benefits and challenges of one New Zealand nursing undergraduate clinical education model: A case study'. From 2006 to 2008, Deborah was a Coresearcher for the CPIT/CDHB Dedicated Education Unit pilot project. More recently (2008–2010), Deborah has been a Coresearcher in a research team 'Evaluating the Quality of Workplace Learning and Undergraduate Student Nurses in Community Settings in New Zealand using the Clinical Learning Environment Supervision & Teacher survey tool (CLES+T)'.

Jane Mountier, BA, was employed by Christchurch Polytechnic Institute of Technology (CPIT) as a Research Assistant from 2009 to 2011. She gained her research skills working with nurses who are passionate about nursing education.

The following people, whilst not writing Chapter 6, provided support to Michelle, Deb and Jane.

Dr **Isabel Jamieson**, RN, BN, MNurs (Melb), CertAT, Ph.D., is currently employed by the Christchurch Polytechnic Institute of Technology (CPIT) School of Nursing as a Senior Nursing Lecturer. She is a member of the CPIT and Canterbury District Health Board (CDHB) Dedicated Education Unit Advisory Team and Governance Group. Isabel was a Coresearcher for the CPIT/CDHB Dedicated Education Unit pilot project (2006–2008) and a member of a research team 'Evaluating the Quality of Workplace Learning and Undergraduate Student Nurses in Community Settings in New Zealand using the Clinical Learning Environment Supervision & Teacher survey tool (CLES+T)' for use in hospital and community settings in New Zealand (2008–2010).

Rose Whittle, RN, MEd (Dist), BA (Ed.), Adv. DipN (CP), Cert. Adult Tchg, is a member of the CPIT/Canterbury District Health Board (CDHB) Dedicated Education Unit (DEU) Working and Governance Groups. She has over 25 years' nursing education experience and is Clinical Manager for the School of Nursing at Christchurch Polytechnic Institute of Technology (CPIT). Rose plans clinical experiences for students from the Bachelor of Nursing, Diploma of Enrolled Nursing and Competency Assessment Programmes and individual programmes for Registered Nurses wanting to change their scope of practice. She was a Coresearcher for the DEU pilot project (2006–2008), Independent Evaluator for the Manukau Institute of Technology (MIT)/Counties Manukau District Health Board (CMDHB) Dedicated Education Unit action research project (2009) and a member of the 'CLES+T' research team (2008–2010).

Raylene Shaw, Postgraduate Diploma Hlth Sc, has been a Nurse Educator in General Surgery at Christchurch Hospital, Canterbury District Health Board (CDHB) since 2005. She is a member of the CDHB Dedicated Education Unit Governance Group.

Debbie Cook, RN, Cert Clin Tchg, is an MN Lecturer and Clinical Coordinator for the Department of Nursing and Human Services at Christchurch Polytechnic Institute of Technology (CPIT). Deb is also a Senior Clinical Lecturer in theory and clinical courses and an active member of the Dedicated Education Unit Working and Governance Group.

Teresa Kilkenny, RN, Postgraduate Diploma (Nursing), is a Nurse Educator, Respiratory and General Medicine, Christchurch Hospital, Canterbury District Health Board (CDHB). Teresa is a member of DEU Working Group.

Chapter 8

Margaretha Ekebergh, RN, Ph.D., is a Professor in Caring Science/Caring Science Didactics, School of Health Sciences, Borås University, and Guest Professor at Linnaeus University in Växjö, Sweden. She has extensive experience in nursing practice and teaching in nurse and specialist nurse education, Master's programmes and doctoral studies. Margaretha's research concerns learning in an educational and caring context, focusing on how reflection impacts the intertwining of health-care theory with best practice. She aims to create a deeper understanding for the patient's needs and situation by developing forms of didactics that optimise learning in the health-care sector through innovative environments that bridge the theory-practice gap and promote interaction between caring and learning, based on lifeworld theory and caring science. The Dedicated Education Unit (DEU) was developed within this framework at the Southern Älvsborg Hospital (SÄS), Borås, Sweden. Margaretha is researching the intertwined processes of caring and learning in DEUs in psychiatric care and orthopaedic care.

Chapters 1, 9, 10, 11 and 12

Margaret Bowden, BA, BALibSt (Flinders), is an Editor who is currently a research assistant in the School of Nursing and Midwifery, Flinders University, Adelaide, South Australia. Margaret has worked as a Research Assistant and Editor on varied research projects and publications in Social Sciences, Health Sciences, Education and Engineering over the past 17 years, many of which have focused on work-integrated learning. She has also tutored in Aboriginal Education and works with higher degree students for whom English is not their first language. Margaret is passionate about learning, language and culture.

Chapter 10

Elaine Horn is a Lecturer at Manukau Institute of Technology (MIT), New Zealand, and an Academic Liaison Nurse (ALN) in an MIT Dedicated Education Unit (DEU) in a medical ward in a public hospital in Auckland, New Zealand.

Sheona Watson is a Senior Lecturer/Clinical Coordinator, Nursing and Health Studies, Manukau Institute of Technology, New Zealand. She was a member of the Manukau Institute of Technology (MIT)/Counties Manukau District Health Board (CMDHB, now called Counties Manukau Health) Dedicated Education Unit (DEU) Action Research Group set up in 2009 to evaluate the establishment of two MIT/CMDHB Inpatient DEUs. This role involved coordinating day-to-day operational issues within the Dedicated Education Unit areas, monitoring student/staff satisfaction, facilitating staff communication regarding the processes in place, providing feedback and support to areas and participating in action research.

Anj Taylor and **Vandhana Nand** were 3rd year students at Manukau Institute of Technology (MIT), New Zealand, when they contributed their story to this book. They had come to nursing as a profession after working in very different non-nursing environments. Anj had been an Executive Chef, working in a fast-paced, people-driven, communication-oriented environment in London. Vandhana had been working in a diagnostic lab, isolated from much communication with other people. Both were so inspired by the Dedicated Education Unit (DEU) concept that they applied, with a sense of privilege, to be part of the Manukau DEU, and were keen to share their experiences.

Jen Little-Reece, RN, BSN, is currently an RN at the Providence Portland Medical Center, Portland, Oregon. At the time of her contribution to this book, Jen was a Nursing Student at the University of Portland, Oregon.

Peter Mason, ‘the clinician who is passionate about the DEU’, is currently Safety, Quality and Risk Management Coordinator, Division of Surgery, The Queen Elizabeth Hospital, Adelaide, South Australia. Peter was the Clinical Nurse Consultant (CNC) in the first Dedicated Education Unit at Flinders Medical Centre, South Australia. Peter finished his 3-year hospital-based nursing training in the early 1980s before undertaking a Diploma in Applied Science, Bachelor of Nursing and Master of Nursing. His involvement in Dedicated Education Units occurred whilst he was a

Clinical Nurse Consultant (CNC) of the GI Service/Liver Transplant Unit at Flinders Medical Centre, South Australia.

Ann Harrington, RN, BNg, Ph.D., is a Senior Lecturer and Clinical Researcher, School of Nursing and Midwifery, Flinders University with 33 years' clinical and teaching experience in health and higher education institutions in New South Wales and South Australia. She is passionate about clinical practice and for 6 years was involved in setting up Dedicated Education Units (DEUs) in South Australia. Ann believes the DEU is the best model for melding students' theory and practical skills because it provides the most supportive environment for the students and academic and clinical staff in developing future nurses. She currently teaches qualitative research design, palliative care and spirituality to students in undergraduate and postgraduate programmes. Ann's research interests are in patients', relatives' and health-care providers' views of end-of-life care; spiritual care for older people; the role of the community palliative care nurse; and Registered Nurses' perceptions of spiritual care.

Cathy Andrew, RN, BA, MA (Hons), Ph.D., is Head of the School of Nursing and Human Services at Christchurch Polytechnic Institute of Technology (CPIT), New Zealand. Her practice background includes surgical, mental health and intensive care nursing in New Zealand and the UK. She has been involved in nursing education for the past 18 years and has been Head of School since 2000. Cathy has been involved in teaching and developing pre- and post-registration nursing programmes and supervision of Ph.D. students. She is a Nursing Council auditor and works with a number of education providers as a professional consultant or external adviser.

Mary Gordon is the Executive Director of Nursing for the Canterbury District Health Board (CDHB), New Zealand. As part of the Executive Management Team, she provides advice to the Board and management on clinical governance and clinical/nursing standards. Mary also provides strategic leadership and professional support for nursing and clinical staff working in the Canterbury Health System. Mary has held a number of senior nursing leadership positions over the last 15 years and has been in her current role since 2002.

Tracey Duggan is the Clinical Nurse Consultant (CNC) of an acute medical ward Dedicated Education Unit (DEU) at the Canberra Hospital. She has been Clinical Nurse Consultant since 1989 with the ward constantly changing specialties. It is now a 32-bed Respiratory/Endocrinology/Cardiology and Rheumatology ward. Tracey became involved with DEUs in 2006 and found the challenge of integrating students into the ward in increased numbers across all year groups exciting and beneficial to the students and the ward staff. Tracey trained at Woden Valley Hospital and has worked in medical nursing, aged care, emergency department and management in positions including Nurse Manager, Bed Manager, Director of Nursing for Medical services and Assistant Director of Nursing for the Division of Medicine. Tracey has undertaken 'Practice Development Master Classes' and is a 'Respecting Patients' Choices' Consultant and Trainer.

Thimitra Panteleon graduated from the University of Canberra in 2008. She has worked as an RN at the Canberra Hospital, Australian Capital Territory, Australia, between overseas travel. Thimitra is currently undertaking her Critical Care Graduate Diploma and has a particular interest in supporting families through the patient care journey.

Amanda Husslebee, RN, BNg, completed her Bachelor of Nursing at the University of Canberra in 2007 and worked at the Canberra Hospital from 2008 to 2010. She did her first placement as a new graduate on the Cardiac/Endocrine/Respiratory medical ward (6A, which is a Dedicated Education Unit [DEU]), the same ward on which she had done her final student placement the previous year. Amanda believes going back to a ward with which she was familiar helped her greatly during her transition from student to Registered Nurse. She strongly recommends that other student nurses consider doing this as part of their new graduate programmes. Amanda is currently in the UK, broadening her horizons and conquering the National Health Service (NHS). She believes she would never have had the confidence to do this if it had not been for the support and love she received from her colleagues on DEU Ward 6A.

Marina Boogaerts, DEU Liaison Nurse, ACT Health Community Health DEU, and Clinical Nurse Consultant (CNC), ACT Health Community Health Continuing Care Programme, is an Adjunct Professional Associate—Community Health with the School of Health Sciences at the University of Canberra, ACT, Australia. Marina has worked as a nurse in a variety of settings in Belgium, Switzerland and Australia since completing her nursing studies in Belgium. She has been in a senior nursing role in Australia since 1987 and has worked as a clinical nurse in Australian Capital Territory (ACT) hospitals and in community health. In 2006, her work with students and her contribution to student learning was recognised with an ACT Nursing and Midwifery 'Educational Excellence Award'.

Kylie Finlay and **Paul Griffith** were members of the original pilot Flinders University Dedicated Education Unit at Flinders Medical Centre (FMC), South Australia. Kylie graduated from Flinders University, Adelaide, South Australia, in 1993 and completed the Graduate Nurse Programme at FMC in 1994. She has worked on the GI Unit for 16 years and has been the unit's Clinical Service Coordinator since 2005. Paul Griffith, who had been an RN for approximately 19 years when the first trial Dedicated Education Unit began in 1997 in the GI Unit, was the first Dedicated Education Unit's Liaison Nurse (LN).

Beverley McClelland is the Nurse Leader, Nursing Professional Development Unit (NPDU) at Counties Manukau District Health Board (CMDHB), who for the past 10 years has had a joint appointment with the University of Auckland in the School of Nursing, contributing to curriculum development, course delivery and assessment for postgraduate nursing degrees. Bev has a Master's Degree in Health Science exploring the 'Critical Factors that Influence Staff Retention in an Acute Perioperative Environment'. She places importance on leadership and professional growth and development. Bev leads a team of Nurse Educators/Coordinators and

Clinical Coaches who are quality focused, skilled practitioners performing a crucial role in facilitating effective learning and professional development for all nurses and inter-professionally across the continuum of care. The NPDU team supports students to link practice and theory and acts as catalysts for learning. Bev also manages mentoring and coaching, providing organisational support systems.

Chapter 1
Introduction

Kay Edgecombe and Margaret Bowden

The challenge for nurse educators is 'how best to prepare students for the complexities of the social, cultural and political arena of clinical practice' (Newton et al. 2009: 630). In rising to this challenge, nurse educators have leapt onto the treadmill of innovation, experimentation, evaluation and re-innovation. Powering this treadmill is the question: *How can we do it better?*

The quest to do it better led to a move in the USA in the 1920s, in the UK in the 1980s and in Australia, New Zealand and Sweden in the 1990s to teach nursing jointly in universities and hospitals. This shift from a practice-based model of learning to a more balanced model of learning theory and practice together moved nursing from a *vocation* to a *profession*. The intention was to facilitate a two-way interchange of theory and practice to constantly inform change or adapt to it and to maintain skill and knowledge currency among nurses and academics. Emphasis shifted towards developing students' critical thinking and clinical decision-making skills, a collaborative approach to learning, encouraging research and working whilst learning essential technical nursing skills, the 'whole domain of professional knowledge and practice' (Benner et al. 2010: 25–26), with a focus on teaching for 'a sense of salience' in the clinical context (Benner et al. 2010: 82).

The transition to this dual-site, dual-knowledge integrated learning model for nursing created tensions between health-care organisations (referred to here as 'hospitals' or 'health services') and tertiary education institutions (referred to here as 'universities'). These were essentially tensions between *our* knowledge and ways

K. Edgecombe (✉) • M. Bowden
School of Nursing and Midwifery, Flinders University, GPO Box 2100, Adelaide, SA, Australia, 5001
e-mail: kay.edgecombe@flinders.edu.au; margaret.bowden@flinders.edu.au; margaret.bowden@internode.on.net

K. Edgecombe and M. Bowden (eds.), *Clinical Learning and Teaching Innovations in Nursing*, Innovation and Change in Professional Education 10,
DOI 10.1007/978-94-007-7232-8_1, © Springer Science+Business Media Dordrecht 2014

of doing things and *their* knowledge and ways of doing things (Andrews et al. 2006; Newton et al. 2009) and tensions between *why change* and the *need to change* to meet the demands of a changing world.

Once the transition from hospital-based to university- and hospital-based nurse education had occurred, 'How can we do it better?' became a quest for change. It was time to work together for the common goal of maximising students' clinical learning, university/hospital collaboration and clinical teacher currency and satisfaction (Magnusson et al. 2007), whilst minimising university/hospital tensions (Andrews et al. 2006), economic issues (Wellard et al. 2000), clinical and academic staff burnout (Henderson et al. 2006b), risk to patients (Henderson et al. 2006a) and student dissatisfaction (Curtis et al. 2007).

The Dedicated Education Unit (DEU) is among the latest developments in this quest. Originating from Flinders University School of Nursing, Adelaide, Australia,[1] in 1997 (Edgecombe et al. 1999; Gonda et al. 1999; Wotton and Gonda 1999), the DEU is now emerging globally as a successful conceptual model for work integrated learning within the health-care sector. Over the past decade, nurse educators in Australia, New Zealand, the USA and Sweden have adopted and adapted the DEU as a sustainable, agile clinical teaching and learning strategy.

What Is a Dedicated Education Unit?

Dedicated education units (DEUs) have been defined variously as:

- 'Existing health care units that are further developed through strategic collaboration between nurse-clinicians and academics' (Edgecombe et al. 1999: 166)
- 'Client unit[s] developed into an optimal teaching/learning environment through the collaborative efforts of nurses, management, students and faculty' (Moscato et al. 2007: 32)
- 'Dedicated hospital units in which staff nurses and nursing faculty take on new educational roles to deliver more efficient and effective clinical instruction to nursing students' (RWJF 2012)
- 'An approach intended to give students a more effective and richer clinical experience, make better use of existing resources, allow for the clinical education of increased numbers of students with existing faculty, and bridge the academic and practice communities in ways that benefit both the teaching and patient-care missions' (Warner 2010)
- 'A collaboration among administrators, nurse-clinicians and faculty to create an optimal and efficient learning environment for students' (Warner 2010)
- 'An approach built on a new level of collaboration between nursing schools and hospitals. … staff nurses in a hospital unit become primary instructors for nursing students during clinical rotations, and nursing school faculty serve as mentors and teaching resources for the nurses' (RWJF 2012)

[1] Now the Flinders University School of Nursing and Midwifery.

- 'A caring science learning environment where caring and learning are united in reflective tutoring to support the nursing students' learning process in terms of integrating theory with caring practice and their professional development' (Ekebergh 2007)
- 'A small community where everyone (students, clinicians and academics) is continually learning from each other' (Judy Gonda, Chap. 10, this volume)

It must be stressed that the DEU is a response to varied clinical learning environments and curriculum imperatives. *Flexibility*, or *agility*, is a keystone of the DEU, enabling it to manifest in a variety of ways in accordance with the 'context of the clinical learning opportunities available', for example, in 'acute medical and surgical areas, community service organisations or mental health' (Edgecombe and Bowden 2009: 92). Factors impacting the DEU structure include hospital and university policy, regulators, organisational practice and ethos, staffing levels, funding levels, ward sizes, geographical location and individuals who determine ward and health service cultures. In a 28-bed hospital ward, for example, a DEU may consist of ten 3rd year students commencing placement in week 2 of semester for 2 days a week for 12 weeks; ten 2nd year students commencing placement in week 6 for 2 days a week, attached to the 3rd year students for 10 weeks; and twelve 1st year students (in two consecutive groups of 6) having a placement for 2 days a week from week 10, attached to 2nd year students for 3 weeks per group. This is elaborated and presented in graphic form in Chap. 2 (see Fig. 2.1).

Guiding Principles of Dedicated Education Units

Whilst the physical structure of DEUs must flex to meet the needs of specific clinical contexts and to operate within available resources, all DEUs are based on the following principles:

- Clinicians and academics stand alongside each other and acknowledge each other's strengths—clinicians are expert practitioners; academics are expert educators.
- Relationships between the two built on mutual trust, respect and open communication.
- Clinicians and academics, through close relationships, create a strong, collaborative, collegial partnership between the health service, clinical placement venue and university.
- Collaborative learning and teaching with academics, clinicians and students.
- Preparation—all involved know their roles, responsibilities and actions.
- Ongoing academic and clinical practice development for academic and clinical staff (capacity building) and students.

These principles aim to generate a sense of belonging in clinical environments for students and academic and clinical staff.

A Sense of Belonging in Dedicated Education Units

It is known that 'human beings are fundamentally and pervasively motivated by the need to belong' (Levėtt-Jones et al. 2009), and that a sense of belonging is a vital ingredient for successful practice learning (Edgecombe and Bowden 2009; Hale and Jamieson 2009; Levett-Jones and Lathlean 2008; Newton et al. 2009; Ranse and Grealish 2007). The DEU principles, which are in accord with the DEU's pedagogical basis, create respectful learning environments in which increasingly diverse students, clinicians and academics develop a sense of belonging as valued, equal members of a caring and learning team participating in collaborative learning and teaching. This environment appears well suited to acknowledging and valuing the increasing numbers of international students and nurses who may otherwise experience isolation, stereotyping and loss of confidence in clinical practice settings (Edgecombe et al. 2013). The principles address the issues of lack of peer support and anxiety arising from students' uncertainty about their ability, which Melincavage (2011: 787) identifies as arising from feelings that clinical staff are inconsiderate of students' inexperience, demean the students, abandon them and expose their weaknesses to other staff and students.

In DEUs, clinical staff consider academics and students as contributors to the overall clinical care environment; they are not viewed as visitors or unwanted distractions. Strategies such as badges designating individuals' roles within their DEUs (New Zealand), providing dedicated education space and resources (including texts and computers) and having staff request, welcome and attend student presentations (USA) heighten a sense of belonging and professional identity.

The Pedagogical Approach in Dedicated Education Units

The DEU concept lies in the tenets of practice learning communities (Wenger 1998; Wenger et al. 2002), learning as an experiential, social activity (Dewey 1938; Wenger 2000), situated learning (Lave and Wenger 1991) and adult learning (Brundage 1980; Knowles 1990). The university and health-care settings in which students undertake clinical placements form a close partnership in which they share a mutual vision, goals, respect, understanding of the academic and practice curricula, clear roles and responsibilities, resources, collaboration and clear, honest communication. Learning and learners are valued whether they be hospital- or university-trained students or teachers, clinicians, administrators or other staff who become part of the DEU learning process.

The primary focus is on students, as adults, transforming 'knowledge, skills, strategies and values through experience' (Brundage 1980: 5) and reflection on and in practice (Boud and Walker 1990; Boud et al. 1985; Kolb 1984; Schön 1983, 1987). This transformation is achieved through 'active learning', in which students participate 'in constructing and controlling the language and activities of [their] learning' (Habermas in Carr and Kemmis 1986: 149), and peer learning and teaching. What the student brings to the experience is acknowledged as important (Cooper et al. 2010; Edgecombe and Bowden 2009).

All DEUs are designed to increase students' intentional and incidental clinical learning by immersing them in the academic and practice curricula. DEUs provide students with more quality time in the clinical setting and ongoing intentional guidance from clinical and academic staff. Students are afforded the time and support to personally bond with staff members who invest in these future nurses' education and well-being. DEUs also enable students from different year levels to learn nursing practice together over an extended time, encouraging peer learning and teaching. Peers, all staff in the clinical setting and patients to a lesser extent guide students incidentally in a collaborative learning relationship.

The DEU pedagogical approach creates an environment in which students are encouraged and supported to learn nursing practice, clinical staff are supported in teaching the students and academic staff are supported to spend time in the DEU. Students, academics and clinical staff share the ongoing development and maintenance of clinical and academic skills, and teaching and learning strategies. Academics and clinicians become learners as well as teachers, participating in formal and informal staff capacity building activities provided by the university and the health-care organisation. Workshops attended by academic and clinical staff together, for example, enhance a sense of collegiality. Throughout this book, staff capacity building is implicit in discussions about 'preparation' for the DEU, 'staff development' and 'faculty development'.

The Dedicated Education Unit Difference: Why Do We Need It?

Reviewing the current international literature (2005–2012) related to clinical teaching and learning and clinical learning environments, Kay Edgecombe and Margaret Bowden found that many of the issues that precipitated the conception and inception of the first DEU at Flinders University in 1997 continue to be a source of frustration and innovation today. There is general consensus about the importance of clinical practice experience for student nurses (Perli and Brugnoli 2009), but methods for achieving this with optimal outcomes for the long-term future are varied and contested. Challenges identified when structuring clinical learning placements for student nurses include:

- Achieving a balance between student-centred learning, patient-centred care and resource-centred university and hospital management
- Quality clinical teaching and learning (Emerson 2007; Gaberson and Oermann 2007; Kelly 2007)
- Providing appropriate guidance and supervision to each student (Ironside and McNelis 2010)

- Teaching students to 'think on their feet' and make clinical judgements (Ironside and McNelis 2010)
- A supportive clinical learning environment that engenders a sense of belonging in students (Andrews et al. 2006; Edgecombe and Bowden 2009; Hale and Jamieson 2009)
- Good communication between universities and hospitals
- Valuing of university knowledge by hospital-trained clinical staff and of clinical expertise by universities
- The need for institutional policy (both university and hospital) that includes clinical teaching and supervision in academic and clinical staff workloads

Much of the research undertaken to seek answers to these challenges focuses on students' perspectives of their clinical teachers. The research emphasises the importance of clinical teachers who demonstrate a good understanding of the 'concepts and theories related to patient care in the clinical setting', help students to use these to 'better understand the patients' health problems and care' and 'demonstrate clinical skills and judgement' whilst guiding 'students in developing essential clinical competencies' (Gaberson and Oermann 2007: 47).

Kelly (2007: 886) identifies the qualities of 'the best clinical teachers' as having 'sound interpersonal skills', 'clinical competence' and the 'ability to provide feedback'. They 'know how to teach', are 'good role models' and 'encourage mutual respect' (Kelly 2007). Johnson-Farmer and Frenn (2006: 267) found that teachers' description of their practice matched what students in other studies identified as the qualities they expect from clinical teachers. Faculty need to 'clearly communicate expectations and outcomes', 'use multiple teaching strategies', be 'current and knowledgeable', 'student centred' and able to 'draw all students into active questioning and learning' to make the 'process of discovery enjoyable' (Johnson-Farmer and Frenn 2006). Thus, it is essential to ensure that all clinical teachers (academics and clinicians) are well prepared for their role and maintain a high standard of teaching. This requires initial and ongoing staff capacity building, which is a keystone of the DEU philosophy (see Chap. 9, Edgecombe and Bowden, this volume).

The DEU, which is essentially student centred, builds in consideration of what students bring to the clinical learning environment. Hence, the importance in the DEU philosophy of preparing students effectively for their clinical placement experiences, with a major focus on thorough pre-placement orientation to the clinical setting.

Kay Edgecombe critiqued past and current clinical teaching and learning models to compare them with the DEU (see Table 1.1). She found that the same clinical practice learning concerns that precipitated the original DEU persist today despite innovations implemented to address them (Edgecombe 2005; Edgecombe and Bowden 2009; Edgecombe et al. 1999; Emerson 2007; Gaberson and Oermann 2007; Grealish and Carroll 1998; Gonda et al. 1999; Jamieson et al. 2008; Henderson et al. 2006b; Moscato et al. 2004, 2007; Wotton and Gonda 1999, 2004).

Table 1.1 Critique of clinical learning models

Model	Advantages	Disadvantages	Strategies to address disadvantages
TRADITIONAL MODEL/ BLOCK Academic faculty provide direct supervision for a group of students (8-10) on-site. Usually block of a period of three or more weeks for four or more days per week. *Edgecombe (2005), Emerson (2007), Gaberson and Oermann (2007)*	Teacher has maximum control over the learning and evaluation - can assist students use concepts and theories learned off-site as well as on-site; can select clinical activities that best meet student needs, and course goals and objectives Faculty present skills and concepts as desired, guiding students' thinking and action - accuracy and thoroughness Direct supervision and instruction provides faculty with information for the best possible feedback to students	Students often placed in different areas of a hospital - academic spends time going around areas, may only spend 45 mins a day with each student - teacher not accessible to students when needed Teacher may not be up to date with, or expert in clinical skills, teaching procedures or use of technologies – may be lack of congruence between lecture content and clinical application Time commitment onerous; faculty have other duties such as research, administration and other teaching Teachers are outsiders to the clinical setting - may not understand particular settings, culture or care systems Skills performance may be limited to a set number and type of skills each day, or for each group of students Faculty may determine specific level of performance of specific skill as adequate for independent practice, but rely on staff nurses to provide skill supervision Written work primary source of evaluating students' understanding and application of theory	Change student/patient assignment patterns so students are assigned to care for one patient, with each student responsible for different aspects of care Have full-time faculty orient part-time faculty so they understand how their course relates to the overall curriculum Faculty must work closely with clinical managers and staff to ensure students get effective clinical experience

(continued)

Table 1.1 (continued)

Model	Advantages	Disadvantages	Strategies to address disadvantages
FACULTY-DIRECTED, INDEPENDENT EXPERIENCES MODEL No direct supervision. Students function according to specifically delineated instructions Generally used in community-based settings distant from faculty, who make periodic site visits *Emerson (2007), Gaberson and Oermann (2007)*	Gives students diverse range of experiences	Distance from faculty supervision	Provide clear direction to students to assure student accountability and enable evaluation of their learning Clearly state purpose, prepare students and clinical site, lay down clear directives for tasks and post-task reflection

PRECEPTORSHIP MODEL Long-term student/staff preceptor team One on one clinical supervision – student works alongside preceptor *Edgecombe (2005), Emerson (2007), Gaberson and Oermann (2007), Grealish and Carroll (1998), Jamieson et al. (2008)*	Students work closely with a clinical expert – share perceptions of their learning needs and of their experience – can hear expert nurses articulate the clinical learning process Consistent one to one relationship – opportunity for the student to work with a role model to promote socialization Students develop self-confidence and improve critical thinking and decision-making skills Learn new skills under expert guidance Students responsible for own learning Provides psychosocial support for students - most positive social climate Students part of team/valued Students taught current practice Students adapt more easily to realities of practice	Teaching may be delegated to clinical staff who lack clinical teaching skills – preceptors have inadequate preparation Clinical staff may be unfamiliar with academic curriculum; often lack formal qualifications Lack of consistent Clinical Lecturer Faculty need to 'precept the preceptor' – but not on site during clinical - no dedicated on-site support person Preceptors may receive little preparation for their role Lack of integration of theory, research and practice Individual preceptors responsible for facilitating students' learning – lack of flexibility in assigning students to other preceptors if necessary Time demands on preceptors-increased workloads; difficulties of nurses taking on this role in addition to other duties - burnout Clinical assessment completed by preceptor and Clinical Lecturer (no input from ward staff) Preceptor role and responsibilities may not be clearly defined Clinical Lecturer allocated students across hospital – little time with students Preceptors can feel isolated from University faculty	Consistent Clinical Lecturer who becomes familiar with the practice area More than one Clinical Lecturer – maybe one for each section of hospital that has students so can give more time to those students, rather than one rushing all over the place with limited time to spend with students
ROLE MODELING For first year students *Edgecombe (2005)*	Allows nursing students to observe direct care, discover values related to good and bad aspects of care and discover attributes of nurses that contributed to these Helps students recognize creativity and flexibility in practitioners.	Role models must be committed to the profession, teaching and learning practice must be based on sound knowledge and skills must be an open and approachable communicator – generate good relationships with others If these qualities missing, negative experience for students	Careful selection of role models needed – this may be easier said than done due to time and placement availability constraints

(continued)

Table 1.1 (continued)

Model	Advantages	Disadvantages	Strategies to address disadvantages
FACILITATION/ CLUSTER MODEL One RN to 8 students scattered across several wards *Edgecombe (2005)*		Facilitator may not be familiar with hospital or ward routines, policies and procedures Geographically difficult to give all students enough time, i.e. clinical facilitators not available when needed by students	
PEER TEACHING Second and third year students teach first year students *Edgecombe (2005), Edgecombe et al. (1999), Gonda et al. (1999), Grealish and Carroll (1998), Jamieson et al. (2008), Wotton and Gonda (1999, 2004)*	Helps first year nursing students understand value of the content of first year curriculum when they observe the second year nursing students in clinical practice. Students more inclined to ask questions of peers – less worry about being judged Second and third year students gain confidence in their own learning – recognize how they have improved their own skills and knowledge. Explaining to first year students helped second and third years clarify their own knowledge base. Develop supportive relationships in clinical	Possibility of mis-knowledge perpetuation	Peer teaching/learning needs to occur in a supervised context

COLLABORATIVE MODELS *Emerson (2007), Gaberson and Oermann (2007)* – CTA, CTP and Clinical educator/paired models	Less resource intensive Shared instructional roles	Clinical staff may have no knowledge of the theoretical foundations of clinical nursing education, teaching/learning strategies and evaluation methods Role models of expert nursing practice may not be experts in light of the above situation	Preparation of clinical staff for teaching students
CTA model (Clinical Teaching Associate model) Acute care setting; aim to provide close student supervision for groups of 8-10 students while freeing academic faculty for other role obligations Staff nurses teach and supervise students	Shared decisions related to learning experiences and assignments Both staff nurses and faculty involved in clinical supervision; faculty hold post-conference with students and CTAs at end of the day	CTA's knowledge of theory and approaches to clinical education Academic institutions need to provide preparation and ongoing education in these areas Lot of paperwork for CTAs Increased workload for CTAs; teaching and supervising students as well as patient care	Prepare CTAs for role with education re academic curriculum Provide CTAs time away from normal nursing duties to spend with students, communicate with academics and complete paperwork
CTA modification - staff nurses assume teaching role for small groups 3-4 students on own unit in **more equal relationship with faculty**	Staff nurse satisfaction – opportunity to learn more about clinical instruction and grow professionally (Hansberger et al. 2000) Saves money		

(continued)

Table 1.1 (continued)

Model	Advantages	Disadvantages	Strategies to address disadvantages
CTP model (Clinical Teaching Partner) Shared management of student group by an academic faculty member and a clinical nurse specialist (CNS); faculty member may have a joint appointment, evenly shared and financed by University and hospital; CNS may have an adjunct faculty appointment, employed on a 'per diem' basis as needed by the University	Shared evaluation Shared organisation of clinical work and time requirements CNS is fully oriented by the academic institution; is a Masters prepared nurse with an academic appointment, with potential to work on collaborative projects, research and publications CNS provides orientation to academic faculty and students re hospital policy and procedures CNS evaluated annually according to academic guidelines Faculty freed to pursue scholarly efforts Faculty deal with only one collaborator in the clinical setting, giving more consistency and better communication Can increase faculty time for supervision and teaching of other students using traditional model while enriching some students' overall learning experiences	Lot of paperwork for CNS Increased workload for CNS; teaching and supervising students as well as patient care What happens if CNS unavailable? Where is consistency in, and continuity of communication?	Provide CNS time away from normal nursing duties to spend teaching and supervising students, communicate with academics and complete paperwork Need more than one designated CNS to ensure some continuity for students – perhaps implement shared CNS role among 2 or 3 CNS

Clinical educator/paired model Students work with clinical educators in pairs; appropriate for specialised student experiences such as critical care or emergency nursing		
Clinical Education Unit All ward staff responsible for students' supervision *Henderson, Twentyman et al. (2006)*	All staff clinically current and familiar with environment All staff orientate and supervise student learning experiences	
Dedicated Education Unit Group of 6-10 students in ward/unit; mixture of first, second and third years on shifts together Over extended period of time (e.g. 2 days per week over 16 weeks) or may be as block	Based on trust, mutual respect, collaboration, relationship-building and adult learning principles Ongoing liaison between clinical and academic staff All staff in unit/ward responsible for facilitating student learning Clearly defined roles and responsibilities	Human factors, e.g. may be communication breakdown among academic and clinical staff

(continued)

Table 1.1 (continued)

Model	Advantages	Disadvantages	Strategies to address disadvantages
Edgecombe (2005), Edgecombe et al. (2000), Gonda et al. (2000), Grealish and Carroll (1998), Jamieson et al. (2008), Wotton and Gonda (1999, 2004)	*Roles: Clinical Liaison Nurse* (CLN) (experienced RN acting as liaison between the clinical setting and the University, and as students' major clinical teacher) provides consistent, accessible on-site support for staff and students for duration of clinical placement; coordinates student learning on day to day basis *Academic Liaison Nurse* (ALN) - consistent in the unit – becomes familiar with practice area, staff and students – offers on-site teaching sessions/research support to staff and students. Consolidated hours for ALN so more time in DEU ALN, CLN and clinical staff complete clinical assessment (supernumerary time provided for CLN to do this) Student orientation to DEU – done jointly by CLN and ALN (supernumerary time for CLN) CLN and DEU staff familiar with curriculum ALN provides support for CLN, and vice versa – shared clinical and academic expertise and support Workshops for CLNs Student peer teaching Engenders sense of belonging to the Unit		

The biggest difference between the DEU and traditional clinical learning models is that in the DEU, the clinical staff become the students' primary teachers, working in partnership with nursing school academics. This shift requires the creation and designation of new roles for clinical, academic and administration staff and students as exemplified throughout Chaps. 2, 3, 4, 5, 6, 7, 8, 9, 10, 11 in this volume. The same and similar roles may have different names in different DEUs. These are clarified in the glossary of terms accompanying each chapter. The DEU focuses on *preparation* and ongoing capacity building (professional development) of those who take on these roles, *preparation* of the clinical workplace to transform it into an optimal learning environment before students enter it and *preparation* of the students to go into it.

The other major difference is that the DEU is more about a whole learning environment rather than a single one-to-one learning/teaching relationship. At risk of sounding contradictory, the multiple one-to-one relationships built between students, clinicians and academics within the DEU environment provide the security to enable students to develop confidence and competence in the clinical setting.

Essentially student oriented, the DEU concept responds to the need for a clinical learning environment that supports all teachers (clinical staff and academics) as well as students in their work and in building strong relationships with each other and with other members of clinical and academic staff. Paramount is providing students time and opportunities for practice and research and valuing them as legitimate members of the nursing team. Similarly, clinical and academic staff must be provided supernumerary status to enable them to put in the time needed to afford students opportunities for learning. Peer learning is an integral, valuable element of this model, as is provision of ongoing constructive feedback and assessment (see Edgecombe and Bowden 2009). There is no gap in relationships or students feeling lost if their designated preceptor is absent—they understand that they can ask another staff member for advice.

The DEU is still very much in the early stages of innovation. We need to nurture and sustain it as a clinical teaching and learning strategy that recognises the clinician's educational role as vital in developing nursing students' professional skills and knowledge and maintains:

- Strategies for student learning that take into account both incidental and intentional learning
- Development of peer teaching and learning relationships as an essential component of the DEU clinical learning environment
- Consideration of nursing students as members of the nursing profession to facilitate their development
- A combined university and professional responsibility to nurture nursing students' professional development
- Clinical supervision by academics who are, and are also perceived to be, clinically and educationally credible to facilitate the integration of theory and practice and act as a solid link between education and practice

- Ongoing collaboration between university and clinical units at all organisational levels
- A safe, supportive, non-judgemental clinical learning environment to facilitate student learning
- Clinical staff who are actively involved in the development and evaluation of their clinical learning unit (adapted from Gonda et al. 1999: 168)

Sustaining a DEU should be self-perpetuating and cyclical where there is a strong academic-practice partnership and nurses go on to become teachers (Mulready-Shick and Flanagan 2012).

Dedicated Education Units as a Solution to Global Issues in Nurse Education and Practice

Global issues affecting best practice models for clinical learning in nursing include the increasing diversity of nursing students; poor clinical teacher preparation; underutilisation of clinical expertise of full-time academic staff; casual employment of teachers; ageing faculty; shortage of nurses and nursing faculty; contention re nurse educator's role; continued theory-practice gap; graduates not 'fit for purpose'; emphasis on mentorship models using 'link teachers' who liaise between university and clinical settings, but have no direct engagement with patient care; and different pedagogical approaches to nursing education in different settings, for example, in classrooms, seminars, skills laboratories and clinical settings (Kelly 2007: 885–886).

Shortage of nurses and nursing faculty is a major driver of innovation in nursing clinical learning models. This has resulted in increased enrolments in nursing worldwide, placing additional demands on all levels of administration. Surprisingly, there is little discussion of this major role. The DEU has the potential to relieve some of the pressures of providing high-quality placements for greater numbers of students in this climate of global nursing staff and faculty shortages, higher nursing student enrolments, greater competition for student placements, high clinical staff turnover and increased academic and clinical staff workloads (Hall 2006; Henderson et al. 2006a; Kelly 2007; Moscato 2009; Moscato et al. 2007; Pappas 2007). It can do so by having several students of differing year levels in a ward at any given time, but unlike the preceptor model or clinical facilitator model in which students stay with one clinical staff member, all clinical staff take responsibility for students on the ward.

Whilst acknowledging that the DEU may not be suitable in all clinical settings because it depends on 'the people and the context', those using DEUs see them as providing a '*win*, *win*, *win* situation; a win for the academics, a win for the students and a win for the clinical staff' (Peter Mason, Story 7, Chap. 10, this volume).

There is mounting evidence of the ineffectiveness of traditional clinical education models in preparing the future nurse workforce, and the effectiveness of DEUs, particularly in recent landmark studies in the USA. In 2009, the US National League for Nursing completed a survey of 2,386 nurse educators representing nurse education institutions across all states. A key finding was the need for advancements in clinical education to overcome the nationwide nursing shortage and address the barriers to effective clinical education such as 'lack of quality sites' and 'faculty qualified to teach on-site' and clinical agency-imposed restrictions on numbers of students (Ironside and McNelis 2010). The increasing uptake of the DEU is due largely to its capacity to transform clinical nursing education by providing high-quality clinical learning for increasing numbers of nursing students in fewer available clinical settings without raising costs, in the process addressing the significant workforce issue of faculty shortages, as identified in a study by the US Institute of Medicine (2010). It also addresses the issues of nurses achieving higher levels of education and training through an improved education system that promotes seamless academic progression and being full partners with physicians and other health-care professionals in redesigning health care in the USA (Institute of Medicine 2010). The DEU's ability to flex according to context, its inbuilt clinician and academic staff capacity building (staff development) and its recognition of the need for students to feel they 'belong' in their clinical learning settings set it apart from more traditional models of student nurse practice education. It has achieved Magnet hospital status in the USA (ANCC 2010a, b).

In addition, the DEU's inherent principles, underlying learning philosophies and physical manifestations in clinical settings, are congruent with the three apprenticeships for professional nursing knowledge and education and four 'essential' shifts in emphasis for integrating classroom and clinical on-site learning and teaching that Benner et al. (2010: 25–26, 82–83) recommend for 'radical transformation' of clinical education. The shift from an emphasis on 'socialisation' to an emphasis on 'formation' in their landmark nursing education study is essentially what the DEU aims to accomplish, the transformation of the whole person to become a professional nurse.

The Robert Wood Johnson Foundation-sponsored *Evaluating Innovations in Nursing* project supported an evaluation of DEUs at the University of Portland and three replication sites in the USA. The findings indicate that the DEU has 'promise in addressing the nurse faculty shortage, strengthening academic-clinical collaborations and improving clinical education outcomes for students' (Nishioka et al. 2012: iii). Much earlier, a Joanna Briggs Institute systematic review of clinical placement models found that DEUs achieve 'a high level of student satisfaction, and improved communication and collaboration between University departments and clinical facilities' (Lockwood 2003: 31).

Whilst these studies bolster the rationale for the use of DEUs in nurse clinical education, the DEU remains underexposed, underutilised and under-researched.

Dedicated Education Units Around the World

DEUs are now operating in Australia, the USA, New Zealand and Sweden. DEUs developed and trialled in *Australia* include the Flinders University DEU model, as already outlined (Edgecombe and Bowden 2009; Edgecombe et al. 1999; Gonda et al. 1999; Wotton and Gonda 1999), and the Canberra University DEU model (Owen and Grealish 2006) based on the Flinders model, and underpinned by communities of practice theory (Wenger 1998). Students are coached by academic staff in the field (Principal Academics), are included as members of the team and actively participate in the ward's work.

The USA is now leading the way with DEU implementation. The University of Portland, Oregon (Moscato 2009), was first to introduce DEUs. It uses staff nurses who want to teach as Clinical Instructors (CI), prepares them for their role through collaborative staff and faculty development activities, uses existing resources and supports professional development of nurses. In the University of Colorado DEUs, students have a 4-week clinical learning experience, and the key role is that of Clinical Scholar, 'an expert clinical nurse who meets the requirements for providing clinical education for nursing students' and acts as a preceptor to new graduate RNs and as a coach to staff preceptors (Pappas 2007: 42). The University of New Mexico Hospital (Wachdorf 2007) has adapted scheduling to provide more clinical placements and 'certain nurses [have been assigned] to work consistently with certain students'. The University of South Carolina/Palmetto Health partnership DEU (Palmetto Health n.d.) uses a registered nurse Clinical Instructor (CI) from Palmetto Health and a Clinical Faculty Coordinator (CFC) from the university, who plans students' experiences and informs the CI what is covered in class each week. The University at Buffalo and Roswell Park Cancer Institute, developed by hospital administrators, nurse clinicians and University at Buffalo faculty as an adaptation of the University of Portland, Oregon model, has specially trained hospital-based nurses who act as staff Clinical Instructors (CI) and share their clinical experience, knowledge and expertise with the student nurses. This model has been evaluated as 'a win-win situation for nursing education and service-practice partners, with the ultimate beneficiaries being the recipients of nursing care in Western New York' (Kemsley in Anzalone 2010). There are also DEU partnerships between the universities of Massachusetts Boston, Johns Hopkins, Tennessee, Mississippi, Idaho and Washington and their collaborating hospitals and health services. In the DEUs at the University of Massachusetts Boston, students and nurses 'emphasize safety and quality competency development' (Mulready-Shick et al. 2009).

In *New Zealand*, the Christchurch Polytechnic Institute of Technology and Canterbury District Health Board collaboration (CPIT/CDHB) DEU model builds on the one-to-one preceptorship model, with a Clinical Liaison Nurse (CLN) and an Academic Liaison Nurse (ALN) working together to ensure students get as many learning opportunities as possible during their clinical placement (Jamieson et al. 2008; Sims 2008). There is also the Manukau Institute of Technology and Manukau Counties District Health Board (MIT/MCDHB) collaborative DEU, which, like the CPIT/CDHB DEU, uses the CLN and ALN model to provide a dynamic learning environment for clinical and academic staff as well as students (Fourie and McLelland 2010). Manukau has undertaken considerable action research into the DEU.

In *Sweden*, at the University of Borås, the DEU has been developed in collaboration with two hospitals (Södra Älvsborgs Sjukhus and Alingsås Sjukhus) and one community (Alingsås kommun). The DEU is seen as scientific with its basis in caring science. A lifeworld perspective is the frame of reference for learning and tutoring (Ekebergh 2007). The DEU is characterised by a reflective approach and has clear strategies for caring and learning as parallel and common phenomena. The DEU concept offers qualified tutoring and active patient care development (Ekebergh and Määttä 2005; Lindahl et al. 2009). DEUs operate in six different clinical settings, which have been adapted and appropriated to the nursing education programme and curriculum. They are dedicated to nursing students and have a profile related to caring science and a lifeworld perspective. They are first and foremost units and contexts for learning but also provide for research and development in caring.

Another university in Sweden, Linnaeus University, has developed a DEU in a modified form with small units—parts of ordinary wards in the hospital and community care settings—adapted to nursing students' clinical training. The profile and tutoring model are the same as at the University of Borås.

This brief overview provides a snapshot of known DEUs as a prelude to full descriptions of several of these in Chaps. 2, 4, 5, 6, 7 and 8 (this volume) and personal stories from students and academic, clinical and administrative staff about their experiences of setting up and learning, teaching and working in DEUs.

Book Structure

This book will take you on a journey through the development of the DEU from its conception and original implementation to global evolution, adaptation and uptake to meet the challenges inherent in nursing students' clinical practice learning in diverse clinical contexts. The different foci of the chapters reflect the differences in DEUs in varied locations, including the use of different terminology to describe academic and clinical staff roles.

Chapter 2 provides the foundation for the rest of the book. It introduces the factors that precipitated the conceptualisation of the DEU at Flinders University, Adelaide, Australia, in the 1990s and details the conceptualisation process, including a critique of nurse education clinical learning models and the development of DEU-specific roles.

Chapter 3 focuses on the DEU as a well-developed community of practice. It provides an historical analysis of the pedagogical imperatives and priorities for nursing education that have generated interest in the DEU. Learning in the workplace is used as a theoretical framework to discuss concepts such as the invitational quality of the learning environment, student agency and the pedagogies of teaching and assessment in clinical education. The value of the social theory of learning—known as community of practice theory—to promote knowledge learnt through experience in the DEU is explored, with questions posed for further research in curriculum design, pedagogy, stakeholder engagement and the DEU as a learning organisation.

Chapters 4, 5, 6, 7, and 8 describe how DEUs have been implemented in different contexts (process), the challenges involved in setting them up and managing them (policy, institutional support, clinical and academic staff capacity building, administration, stakeholder perceptions), timeframes, evaluation, outcomes and future directions.

Chapter 4 explains the piloting, subsequent implementation and evaluation of the original DEU at Flinders University, Adelaide, Australia. It describes how the guiding principles and roles were put into practice and how the outcomes were evaluated. It focuses on the importance of partnership and leadership, particularly in the initial stages of the first pilot DEU, and their continued importance through the second pilot study and implementation of the first fully operational DEUs.

Chapter 5 focuses on the uptake of the DEU by the University of Canberra (UC), Australia. It describes curriculum design, roles and responsibilities, support for student learning, engaging clinicians in the learning culture, assessment and specific ways of structuring DEUs (acute, multisite and distributive models) in specific health service contexts (community, public, private and mental health settings). It also discusses the value of the academic in the clinical learning environment, benefits and challenges of DEUs, and the need for ongoing revision and engagement to further develop DEUs and identify research possibilities.

Chapter 6 describes the transformation of the traditional clinical teaching model at the University of Portland (UP), Oregon, into the American version of the DEU in response to the need to increase the number of graduates to address a shortage of nurses and faculty. This chapter highlights the importance of establishing respectful relationships with clinical partners, the process of creating a new educational experience, lessons learnt in that process and the role DEUs play in the accreditation of clinical partners as Magnet Hospitals, a revered status that is a critical part of the transformation.

Chapter 7 outlines how the DEU has become the preferred model of clinical learning and teaching in Canterbury, New Zealand. It describes the journey of two organisations (Christchurch Polytechnic Institute of Technology and Canterbury District Health Board) working together to strengthen relationships between nursing education and clinical practice and to enhance the clinical learning environment for undergraduate nursing students. Key foci include action research in the DEU, the principles underpinning the collaborative organisational partnership, implementation of the current DEU model in different clinical settings, quality maintenance, evaluation and future directions for DEUs in Canterbury.

Chapter 8 provides a perspective of the DEU as a learning environment in which caring and learning are united in 'reflective tutoring'; great value is placed on the patients' perspective. The chapter discusses the overall purpose and structure of the University of Borås DEU in Sweden, which uses a 'lifeworld perspective' as its frame of reference for learning and teaching (tutoring). The chapter explains the Borås DEU's scientific and philosophical bases, its focus on patient-centred student learning and reflection and research in the DEU. This chapter illustrates the uniqueness of the Borås approach to, and implementation of, their DEU.

Chapter 9 moves away from specific DEUs to discuss academic and clinical staff capacity building strategies (staff preparation for their roles in DEUs and professional development). It focuses on workshops as a key capacity building strategy. Capacity building is also discussed in relation to understanding assessment processes (clinical and academic staff and students), integrating academic and clinical curriculums and building students' teaching and learning capacity through peer teaching.

Chapter 10 presents a series of personal stories from people involved in all roles in the DEUs (students, graduate RNs, clinicians, clinical facilitators, Principal Academics (PA), Liaison Nurses (LN), Clinical Nurse Consultants (CNC), ward managers, heads of nursing and governance group members). It represents the human experience of the benefits and challenges of immersion in setting up or managing a DEU. The voices from DEUs in Australia, New Zealand, the USA and Sweden bear testament to the emotional and physical realities of learning and working in different roles within different DEUs.

Chapter 11 offers the scaffolding on which to build a DEU to suit any clinical context. This chapter draws on the previous chapters to identify and emphasise the key requisites for successful development and implementation of DEUs in different contexts. It revisits partnership, leadership, marketing, research, evaluation, renovation and innovation, proposing that these same building blocks are needed to successfully construct, maintain and sustain any innovation in the context of work integrated learning. The authors detail the Christchurch Polytechnic Institute of Technology/Canterbury District Health Board (CPIT/CDHB) partnership DEU model as a good practice model to illustrate how the DEU process works, from the initial concept to planning, implementation, management, evaluation and sustainability.

The conclusion to the book stresses again that the DEU is not a fixed model but a concept—a philosophy and set of principles that can be applied in different ways to suit different contexts to achieve a premium clinical learning and teaching environment. It summarises the content of all chapters before discussing 'where to next' for DEUs, focusing on increased research and evaluation of DEUs; using DEUs as clinical research resources for students, academics and clinicians; and expanding DEUs to include multidisciplinary learning and teaching teams to encompass the multidisciplinary nature of patient care.

References

American Nurses Credentialing Center. (2010a). *Forces of magnetism*. http://www.nursecredentialing.org/Magnet/ProgramOverview/ForcesofMagnetism.aspx. Accessed 12 Nov 2011.

American Nurses Credentialing Center. (2010b). *Announcing a new model for ANCC's Magnet Recognition Program*. http://www.nursecredentialing.org/Magnet/ProgramOverview/New-Magnet-Model.aspx. Accessed 12 Nov 2011.

Andrews, G., Brodie, D. A., Andrews, J. P., Hillan, E., Thomas, B. G., Wong, J., & Rixon, L. (2006). Professional roles and communication in clinical placements: A qualitative study of nursing students' perceptions and some models for practice. *International Journal of Nursing Studies, 43*, 861–874.

Anzalone, C. (2010). *UB School of Nursing expands its model to ease nursing shortage, promote excellence in clinical nursing education*. http://www.buffalo.edu/news/10875. Accessed 24 May 2010.

Benner, P., Sutphen, M., Leonard, V., & Day, L. (2010). *Educating nurses: A call for radical transformation*. San Francisco: Jossey-Bass.

Boud, D., & Walker, D. (1990). Making the most of experience. *Studies in Continuing Education, 12*(2), 61–80.

Boud, D., Keogh, R., & Walker, D. (Eds.). (1985). *Reflection: Turning experience into learning*. London: Kogan Page.

Brundage, D. H. (1980). *Adult learning principles and their application to program planning*. Queens Park: Minister of Education Ontario.

Carr, W., & Kemmis, S. (1986). A critical approach to theory and practice. In W. Carr & S. Kemmis (Eds.), *Becoming critical: Knowing through action research* (2nd ed.). Geelong: Deakin University Press.

Cooper, L., Orrell, J., & Bowden, M. (2010). *Work integrated learning: A guide to effective practice*. London: Routledge.

Curtis, J., Bowen, I., & Reid, A. (2007). You have no credibility: Nursing students' experiences of horizontal violence. *Nurse Education in Practice, 7*(3), 156–163.

Dewey, J. (1938). *Experience and education*. New York: Simon & Schuster.

Edgecombe, K. (2005). *Nursing students' perceptions of the Dedicated Education Unit as an effective clinical learning environment*. Unpublished master's thesis. Flinders University, Adelaide.

Edgecombe, K., & Bowden, M. (2009). The ongoing search for best practice in clinical teaching and learning: A model of nursing students' evolution to proficient novice registered nurses. *Nurse Education in Practice, 9*(2), 91–101.

Edgecombe, K., Wotton, K., Gonda, J., & Mason, P. (1999). Dedicated Education Units 1: A new concept for clinical teaching and learning. *Contemporary Nurse, 8*(4), 166–171.

Edgecombe, K., Jennings, M., & Bowden, M. (2013). International nursing students and what impacts their clinical learning: Literature review. *Nurse Education Today, 33*(2), 138–142. doi:10.1016/j.nedt.2012.07.015. Epub 2012 Aug 30.

Ekebergh, M. (2007). Lifeworld-based reflection and learning: A contribution to the reflective practice in nursing and nursing education. *Reflective Practice, 8*(3), 331–343.

Ekebergh, M., & Määttä, S. (2005). *Lärandet på en utbildningsvårdsavdelning—att sammanbinda vårdvetenskaplig teori med vårdpraxis* [Learning in an educational unit—Intertwining caring science in theory with caring practices]. Forskningsrapport, Institutionen för Vårdvetenskap: Högskolan i Borås Rapport nr 1 (Research report, Borås: School of Health Care Sciences Borås University).

Emerson, R. J. (2007). *Nursing education in the clinical setting*. St. Louis: Mosby/Elsevier.

Fourie, W., & McLelland, B. (2010). *Research report on completion of the first cycle of the action research*. Auckland: Collaborative Nursing Development Unit, Manukau Institute of Technology and Counties Manukau District Health Board, New Zealand.

Gaberson, K. B., & Oermann, M. H. (Eds.). (2007). *Clinical teaching strategies in nursing* (2nd ed.). New York: Springer.

Gonda, J., Wotton, K., Edgecombe, K., & Mason, P. (1999). Dedicated Education Units 2: An evaluation. *Contemporary Nurse, 8*(4), 172–176.

Grealish, L., & Carroll, G. (1998). Beyond preceptorship and supervision: A third clinical teaching model emerges for Australian nursing education. *Australian Journal of Advanced Nursing, 15*(2), 3–11.

Hale, J., & Jamieson, I. (2009, September 30–October 2). *Dedicated Education Units: Enhancing nurse students' belongingness*. PowerPoint presentation at 'Working together: Education and practice'. Australasian Nurse Educators Conference, Christchurch, New Zealand.

Hall, W. (2006). Developing clinical placement in times of scarcity. *Nurse Education Today, 26*, 627–633.

Henderson, A. J., Forrester, K., & Heel, A. (2006a). The establishment of structures and processes for the safe and effective clinical placement of nursing students. *Nurse Education in Practice, 6*, 275–280.

Henderson, A., Twentyman, M., Heel, A., & Lloyd, B. (2006b). Students' perception of the psychosocial clinical learning environment: An evaluation of placement models. *Nurse Education Today, 26*, 564–571.

Institute of Medicine. (2010). *The future of nursing; Leading change, advancing health*. http://www.iom.edu/Reports/2010/The-Future-of-Nursing-Leading-Change-Advancing-Health.aspx. Released October 5th 2010. Accessed 12 Nov 2011.

Ironside, P. M., & McNelis, A. M. (2010). *Clinical education in prelicensure nursing programs: Results from an NLN National Survey 2009*. New York: National League for Nursing.

Jamieson, I., Hale, J., Sims, D., Casey, M., Whittle, R., & Kilkenny, T. (2008). *Establishing Dedicated Education Units for undergraduate nursing students: Pilot project summation report*. Christchurch: CPIT Publishing Unit.

Johnson-Farmer, B., & Frenn, M. (2006). Teaching excellence: What great teachers teach us. *Journal of Professional Nursing, 25*(5), 267–272.

Kelly, C. (2007). Students' perceptions of effective clinical teaching revisited. *Nurse Education Today, 27*, 885–892.

Knowles, M. (1990). *The adult learner: A neglected species* (Rev. ed.). Houston: Gulf Publishing.

Kolb, D. A. (1984). *Experiential learning: Experience as the source of learning and development*. Englewood Cliffs: Prentice Hall.

Lave, J., & Wenger, E. (1991). *Situated learning: Legitimate peripheral participation*. New York: Cambridge University Press.

Levett-Jones, T., & Lathlean, J. (2008). Belongingness: A prerequisite for nursing students' clinical learning. *Nurse Education in Practice, 8*(2), 103–111.

Levett-Jones, T., Lathlean, J., Higgins, I., & McMillan, M. (2009). Staff and student relationships and their impact on nursing students' belongingness and learning. *Journal of Advanced Nursing, 65*(2), 316–324.

Lindahl, B., Dagborn, K., & Nilsson, M. (2009). A student-centered clinical education unit—Description of a reflective learning model. *Nurse Education in Practice, 9*(1), 5–12.

Lockwood, C. (2003). *The effectiveness of undergraduate clinical placement, models, methods and meaningfulness for key stakeholders in South Australia* (pp. 1–38). Adelaide: Centre for Evidence based Nursing South Australia, The Joanna Briggs Institute.

Magnusson, C., O'Driscoll, M., & Smith, P. (2007). New roles to support practice learning – Can they facilitate expansion of placement capacity? *Nurse Education Today, 27*, 643–650.

Melincavage, S. (2011). Student nurses' experiences of anxiety in the clinical setting. *Nurse Education Today, 31*, 785–789.

Moscato, S. (2009, June 2). *Dedicated Education Unit clinical teaching model*. PowerPoint presentation, 6th Annual Missouri Foundation for Health summit, Health Care Workforce Development—Cultivating Missouri's Resources. Marriott Centre in Town and Country, St. Louis, MO.

Moscato, S. R., Kaakinen, J., Mitchell, C., Gatlin, P., & Miller, J. (2004). Dedicated Education Unit: Innovative strategy for optimal clinical learning. *Communicating Nursing Research, 37*, 247. In Proceedings of 37th annual Communicating Nursing Research Conference; 18th annual WIN Assembly, 'Hallmarks of quality: Generating and using knowledge', 22–24 April, Portland OR.

Moscato, S., Miller, J., Logsdon, K., Weinberg, S., & Chorpenning, L. (2007). Dedicated Education Unit: An innovative clinical partner education model. *Nursing Outlook, 55*, 31–37.

Mulready-Shick, J., & Flanagan, K. (2012). *Project PDQ–Partnering for DEU development and quality.* http://www.evaluatinginnovationsinnursing.org/our-grantees/massachusetts/ Accessed 27 Feb 2013.

Mulready-Shick, J., Kafel, K., Banister, G., & Mylott, L. (2009). Enhancing quality and safety competency development at the unit level: An initial evaluation of student learning and clinical teaching on dedicated education units. *Journal of Nursing Education, 48*(12), 716–719.

Newton, J., Billett, S., & Ockerby, C. M. (2009). Journeying through clinical placements: An examination of six student cases. *Nurse Education Today, 29*, 630–634.

Nishioka, V., Coe, M., Moscato, S., & Hanita, M. (2012, February). *Dedicated education units—Evaluating innovation in clinical education.* Final Technical Report. Supported by a grant from the Robert Wood Johnson Foundation, Evaluating Innovations in Nursing Education National Program Office. www.nursing.up.edu

Owen, J., & Grealish, L. (2006). Clinical education delivery. A collaborative, shared governance model provides a framework for planning, implementation and evaluation. *Collegian, 13*(2), 15–21.

Palmetto Heath. (n.d.). *Palmetto Heath DEU.* http://www.palmettohealth.org/body.cfm?id=3514&oTopID=0. Accessed 24 May 2010.

Pappas, S. (2007). Improving patient safety and nurse engagement with a Dedicated Education Unit. *Nurse Leader, 5*(3), 40–43.

Perli, S., & Brugnoli, A. (2009). Italian nursing students' perception of their clinical learning environment as measured with the CLEI tool. *Nurse Education Today, 29*, 886–890.

Ranse, K., & Grealish, L. (2007). Nursing students' perceptions of learning in the clinical setting of a Dedicated Education Unit. *Journal of Advanced Nursing, 58*(2), 171–179.

RWJF. (2012). *Putting innovations in nursing education to the test. RWJF program funds evaluations of creative new approaches to address the nurse faculty shortage.* http://www.rwjf.org/publichealth/product.jsp?id=56172. Accessed 22 June 2012 (publ. February 26, 2010).

Schön, D. A. (1983). *The reflective practitioner: How professionals think in action.* New York: Basic Books.

Schön, D. A. (1987). *Educating the reflective practitioner.* San Francisco: Jossey-Bass.

Sims, D. (2008). *Destination DEU. Getting started: A New Zealand experience.* PowerPoint presentation to National Nurse Education Conference, Sydney, Australia.

Wachdorf, H. (2007, March 23). UNMH testing new scheduling plan for nursing students. *New Mexico Business Weekly*, Online. http://albuquerque.bizjournls.com/albuquerque/stories/2007/03/26/story10.html. Accessed 6 Nov 2009.

Warner, J. (2010). University of Portland, Oregon. In RWJF (2012). *Putting innovations in nursing education to the test. RWJF program funds evaluations of creative new approaches to address the nurse faculty shortage.* http://www.rwjf.org/publichealth/product.jsp?id=56172. Accessed 22 June 2012.

Wellard, S., Williams, A., & Bethune, E. (2000). Staffing of undergraduate clinical learning programs in Australia. *Nurse Education Today, 20*, 548–554.

Wenger, E. (1998). *Communities of practice: Learning, meaning and identity.* Cambridge: Cambridge University Press.

Wenger, E. (2000). Communities of practice and social learning systems. *Organization, 7*(2), 225–246.

Wenger, E., McDermott, R., & Snyder, W. (2002). *Cultivating communities of practice: A guide to managing knowledge.* New York: Harvard Business School Press.

Wotton, K., & Gonda, J. (1999, July 12–15). *Redesigning clinical experience for undergraduate nursing students: an innovative model.* Paper presented at HERDSA 1999 conference "What do we value in higher education?" Melbourne.

Wotton, K., & Gonda, J. (2004). Clinician and student evaluation of a collaborative clinical teaching model. *Nurse Education in Practice, 4*(2), 120–127.

Chapter 2
Dedicated Education Units in Nursing: The Concept

Kay Edgecombe

Glossary of Terms in Order of Appearance in This Chapter

Clinical lecturer/clinical facilitator academic staff who visit the clinical learning setting intermittently to provide curriculum integration and monitor the student's progress with the student and their preceptor; may also undertake research projects in the clinical setting

Block placement students placed in clinical setting for a short, concentrated block of time, overseen by academic lecturers

Cluster model block placement with one academic lecturer working with a group of students and two RNs

Preceptor model one student allocated to one preceptor (experienced RN)

Hospital-based apprenticeship model students learn from more senior clinical staff in the hospital and from each other

Clinical lecturers academic staff who visit the clinical learning setting intermittently to provide curriculum integration and monitor the student's progress with the student and their preceptor; may also undertake research projects in the clinical setting

Clinical Placement Coordinator (CPC) academic in the School of Nursing responsible for negotiating clinical placements and ensuring placements are congruent with curriculum requirements for the whole undergraduate programme

K. Edgecombe (✉)
School of Nursing and Midwifery, Flinders University, GPO Box 2100, Adelaide, South Australia, Australia, 5001
e-mail: kay.edgecombe@flinders.edu.au

K. Edgecombe and M. Bowden (eds.), *Clinical Learning and Teaching Innovations in Nursing*, Innovation and Change in Professional Education 10,
DOI 10.1007/978-94-007-7232-8_2, © Springer Science+Business Media Dordrecht 2014

Clinical Nurse Consultant (CNC) most senior nurse in the DEU responsible for overall running of the unit

Liaison Nurse (LN) full time Registered Nurse (RN) responsible for overseeing clinical in the DEU

Principal Academic (PA) a permanent School of Nursing lecturer responsible for communicating and liaising with the students, the LN and the CNC and utilising their ongoing expertise to facilitate students' learning

Clinicians Registered Nurses (RNs) and Enrolled Nurses (ENs) recognised as clinician educators for students, responsible for facilitating students' learning in collaboration with the PA and LN

Clinical Placement Officer (CPO) general administrative staff member in the School of Nursing responsible for student placement administrative processes.

Introduction

In writing this chapter, I reflect on my role as the protagonist of the Dedicated Education Unit (DEU) in nursing and as a partner with my academic and clinical colleagues, in particular Judy Gonda, Karen Wotton and Dianne Longson, in bringing the DEU to fruition.

The early 1990s was a period of significant change in workplace organisation in health services and universities in South Australia. Changes in staffing, policy and management combined with budget restraints to heighten stress on clinical and academic staff at a time when they were grappling with the practicalities of the recent shift of nurse education from the hospital-based apprenticeship model to a joint enterprise between the health care sector and the university sector. There were fewer permanent experienced staff in clinical venues and universities. Clinical venues showed heightened resistance to taking students under the placement arrangements used at that time. Students undertaking a standard 3-year undergraduate Bachelor of Nursing degree wanted more time in the practice learning environment, and clinical and academic staff needed more time to teach them while upgrading their own theoretical knowledge and practical skills. These pressures manifested in a negative attitude towards students in clinical contexts. Students became a source of angst or extra pairs of hands rather than being seen as future nurses. The clinical learning environment had become toxic.

The key people involved in nursing students' clinical education were the clinical nursing staff and the students. The clinical nursing staff willingly provided the vast majority of the teaching in the clinical environment; viewed students as important to the profession and the future of nursing; valued their own capacity to demonstrate the knowledge, skills and attitudes of being a nurse; and expressed frustration at not seeing the outcomes of their teaching efforts. Students were in clinical for too

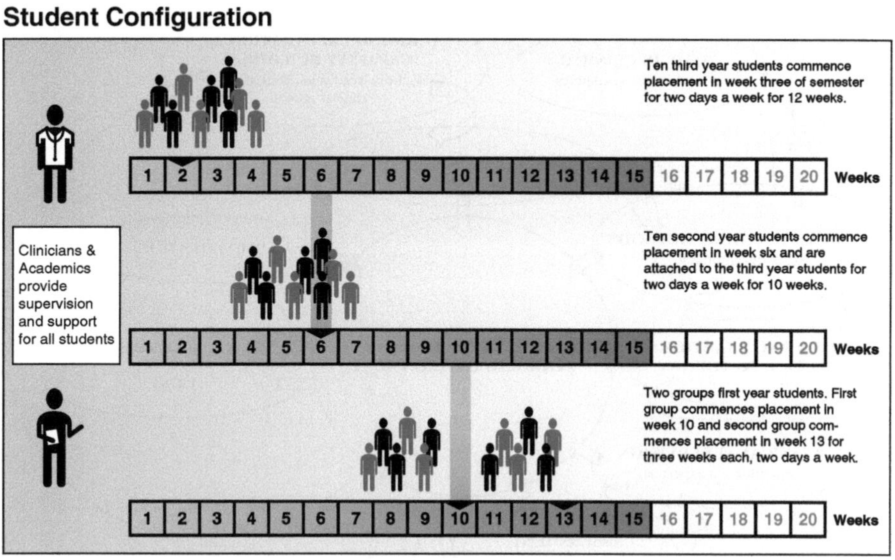

Fig. 2.1 Student configuration in initial Flinders' DEUs

short a time for clinical staff to measure their learning progression or their capacity to perform the nursing role. Yet, clinical placement venues and the university appeared to take for granted the clinical staff's crucial clinical education role. These clinical educators received no feedback on their performance as teachers or on their students' performance, no preparation for teaching the students, no orientation time with the students and no knowledge about the students' curriculum or intended learning outcomes. Nor did they have reliable lines of communication with the university.

A new clinical placement strategy was urgently needed. My colleagues and I believed we had the range of expertise and resources to initiate change. That change took the form of the DEU. The focus here is on the DEU conceptualisation process, not its implementation.

I wish to emphasise that while I conceptualised and initiated the DEU, Judy, Karen and Dianne enthusiastically engaged with its development in preparation for its implementation. Before describing the conceptualisation, it is important to present the student configuration in the application of the initial DEUs, as depicted by Judy Gonda (Fig. 2.1) and provide a 'thought map' illustrating the elements I recognised as having an impact on the DEU as a whole clinical learning environment (see Fig. 2.2). Several colleagues worked with me to develop the concept to a point where we could submit it to the School of Nursing as a proposal for change, after which it was presented to the regional directors of Nursing. The original concept was further finessed by a working party and later by an advisory group. Judy Gonda details these processes in Chap. 4 (this volume), which focuses on the implementation of the original DEU.

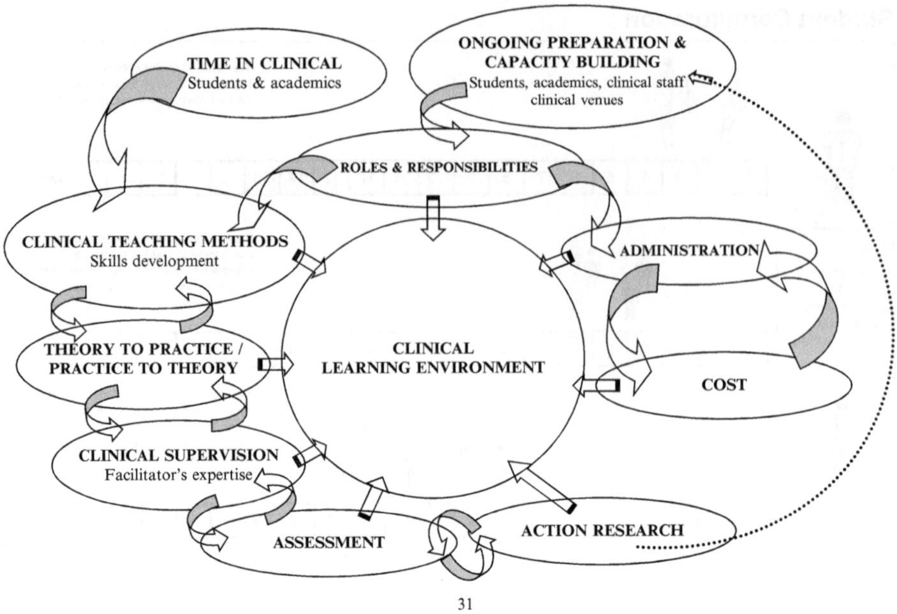

Fig. 2.2 Factors impacting the quality of the clinical learning environment

The Dedicated Education Unit as a Clinical Learning Environment

The primary purpose of the DEU as a clinical education strategy was to understand, value and develop a learning environment in which:

1. Students were active learners—risk takers[1] and confident, competent learners who had quality learning outcomes in a real world setting. They experienced the reality of nursing practice and patient care in an environment in which real patients were central to their learning, giving them the opportunity to draw on their knowledge, skills and values to perform as professionals and to reflect on their learning in a supported, safe learning environment.
2. Clinical staff were expert practitioners and the students' primary teachers.
3. Academics were expert educators who facilitated the students' integration of theory and practice.

The DEU was a ward dedicated to students' clinical education. Ideally, this environment engaged students, clinicians and clinical lecturers in the excitement

[1]Risk takers only in the sense of being prepared to make, and capable of making decisions, and taking appropriate, *safe* action, under appropriate levels of guidance from clinical supervisors; adopting the attitude and developing the competence to progress to autonomous practice.

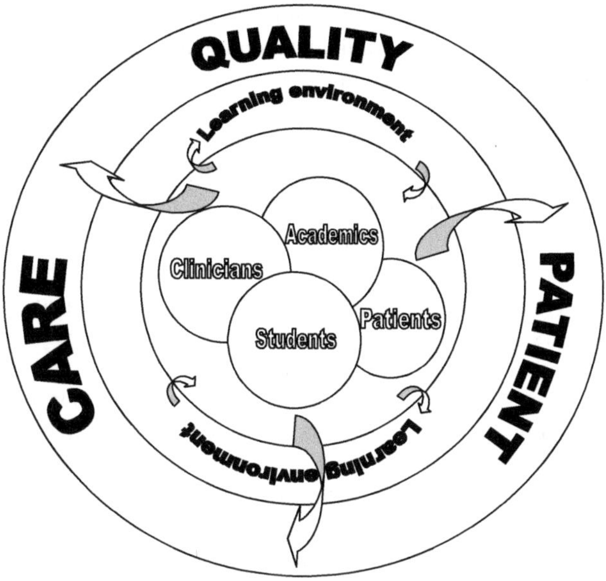

Fig. 2.3 Factors impacting the quality of patient care

of learning through addressing issues previously identified as problematic. It gave students the support they needed to gain a sense of security while having enough autonomy to meet challenges and experience a degree of risk. It provided clinical staff with support from the university and the health service to put time and energy into teaching the students and advancing their own learning.

Importantly, the environment incorporated continuous lines of communication between the clinical venue and the university for students, clinical staff and clinical lecturers. This ongoing connection between the clinical venue and the university was enhanced through a change in the physical structure of clinical placements in DEUs. Only Flinders University nursing students were placed in a DEU, and their placement consisted of 2 days per week throughout the semester rather than a concentrated block of time (see Fig. 2.1).

Figures 2.2 and 2.3 illustrate the factors that built the DEU clinical learning environment and the links between its quality and the quality of patient care.

Conceptualising the Dedicated Education Unit

The aim was, as always as a nurse educator, to develop well-prepared, competent graduates capable of transferring their learning between diverse settings and fulfilling the professional RN role. The search for a clinical learning strategy to achieve this in the turmoil of 1990s' nurse education required synthesising the concerns voiced by clinical educators, students, clinical venue administrators and clinical staff about the current clinical teaching and learning strategies. Issues included difficulties created by having a variety of different students from different years and different institutions coming to each ward with different learning approaches, cultures and objectives; students having no real sense of belonging in the wards, little opportunity to learn through repetition, too little time in their clinical placement and too little opportunity to show they could sustain practice competency; clinical facilitators spread over a wide geographic area within venues and institutions, preventing maintenance of relationships with the clinical nursing staff and currency with their teaching; and difficulties assessing students' progress.

After many years of informal discussions and formal meetings with academic and clinician colleagues and their organisations, research, gathering student feedback and pondering the personal knowledge gained from the hospital training programme as well as practising and teaching nursing, I formed the raw concept of what would become the DEU. It was a clinical placement strategy and whole learning environment that could provide a solution to the resource issues impacting the quality and quantity of student learning in clinical contexts.

Earlier research into collaborative teaching with colleagues Di Longson, Janice Orrell and Judith Gonda from the Flinders University School of Nursing were instrumental in informing the design of the original DEU. The findings clearly established that collaborative teaching had a major influence on students' ability to integrate their learning across the academic and clinical environments (Longson et al. 1997). Therefore, collaborative relationships must form a core element of any new strategy.

Students' major concerns were about not achieving the desired outcomes of their learning, which were competence and recruitment. They related their sense of little consistent or effective interaction in the clinical learning environment and no ongoing assessment of their progress. They did not feel ready to become graduate registered nurses (RNs). It was apparent that there was little collaboration among the institutions and individuals participating in current clinical teaching and learning models.

The concerns that academics, clinical staff and students had expressed were organised into main themes under the headings 'University' (academics), 'Placement Venue' (clinical staff), 'Students' and 'Patients', representing the key collaborators in the intended new strategy (Table 2.1). Quality of patient care was the primary consideration.

The quality of the clinical learning environment became the key focus for achieving high quality patient care. The quality of clinical learning (clinical supervision and level of clinical facilitators' expertise), clinical teaching methods (skills development), teaching informed by practice and theory, length of time in clinical for students and academics, preparation of students, academics, clinicians and clinical venues, roles and responsibilities, assessment, evidence-based research, administration and cost are all strands in the learning environment web. No concern could be addressed separately. Figures 2.2 and 2.3 illustrate the complex relationships among all of the concerns in Table 2.1.

Table 2.1 Main themes re clinical teaching and learning

University	Placement venue	Students	Patients
Classroom environment (theory/practice gap)	Clinical environment (theory/practice gap)	Influence of clinical placement on students (theory/practice gap) Reality shock Impact on patients	Impact on students
Joint appointments	Joint appointments		Quality of care
Clinical supervision	Clinical supervision	Clinical supervision	Quality of care
Clinical teaching methods	Clinical teaching methods	Development of critical thinking skills in practical	Quality of care
Academics' practice role/role in clinical learning	Clinicians' role/role in clinical learning	Students' role/ motivation to learn Resistance	Patient's role—contribution to student learning
Research/evidence-based practice	Research/evidence-based practice	Research/evidence-based practice	Quality of care
Graduate preparation—outcomes (includes clinical skills preparation)	Graduate preparation—outcomes (includes clinical skills preparation)	Graduate preparation—outcomes (includes clinical skills preparation repetition)	Quality of care
	Develop learning environment that will effectively prepare graduates to be RNs	Student mastery Impact on patients	Contribution to student learning
Level of experience of clinical teachers—maintaining practice currency	Level of experience of ward RNs	Quality of learning from RNs	Quality of care
Current practice informing teaching	Education principles informing clinical teaching	Peer teaching	Contribution to student learning
Collegiality—sense of belonging and being valued	Collegiality—sense of belonging and being valued	Collegiality—sense of belonging and being valued	Collegiality—contribution to student learning; sense of being valued
Preparation of academics pre-placement	Preparation of clinical staff and venue pre-placement	Preparation of students pre-placement	Preparation of patients when students on ward—informing patients students will be practising—acceptance, resistance Quality of care

(continued)

Table 2.1 (continued)

University	Placement venue	Students	Patients
Cost: administrative, remuneration	Cost: administrative, remuneration	Cost: loss of income while on placement	
Amount of time in clinical	Amount of time in clinical	Amount of time in clinical—not enough time to practise	Quality of care
Role of dean	Role of director of nursing		Quality of care
Assessment	Assessment	Assessment	Quality of care

Table 2.2 Advantages and disadvantages of models already in use

Hospital	Block	Preceptor	Cluster
Opportunity to learn by repetition[a]	No first-year placement[b]	Student-preceptor relationship—one-to-one; continuity[a,b]	Direct academic and clinical teaching[a]
Peer teaching and learning[a]	Limited to 2–4 students per ward[b]	Feedback on progress[a]	Relationship-building between academic and clinical staff[a]
Collegiality with peers[a]	Only 3 blocks per semester[b]	Resource intense[b]	Intermittent contact and communication[b]
Socialisation and workforce issues taking precedence over teaching and learning[b]	Lack of availability of venues[b]	Unsustainable with numbers of available expert RNs[b]	Dependent on one individual[b]
	Minimal opportunity for peer learning[b]	No opportunity for peer learning[b]	Opportunities for peer learning[a]

[a]Designates advantages
[b]Designates disadvantages/risks

It became essential to generate and support the elements required for the ideal clinical learning environment. These were to support everyone in every role to encourage students; to be enthusiastic and passionate about teaching a new generation of nurses; to be willing to take responsibility for communication and relationship-building; to be generous with their time and knowledge; and to be motivated to make a difference and embrace change. A critique of four clinical teaching and learning placement models used until the mid-1990s in South Australia established what worked well, what did not and why. Each model was critiqued in terms of its advantages and disadvantages. These are summarised in Table 2.2.

This critique led me to a much deeper level of thinking about the design of the DEU.

The cluster model, an earlier clinical placement innovation, unique to our school, was a block-style placement with eight 2nd year students in one ward. It ran over

4 days per week for 3 weeks with a clinical lecturer (academic staff) in situ for the entire shift, every shift and two RNs caring for 16 patients (half the ward). The clinical lecturer and RNs role modelled patient care, but importantly in that context, they evaluated the students' learning and implemented learning strategies specific to individual students.

The cluster model worked effectively for 2nd year students in larger hospitals where the clinical staff and nursing administration regarded it highly, and patients responded positively to the intensive learning support for the students and the attention students gave them. But it did not translate into 3rd year learning and was not viable for 1st year students (who had no placement programme at all at that time). It also became *unsustainable* when the people who had initiated it were no longer directly involved.

The knowledge gained from the critique coupled with my practical experience of all four models impressed on me the necessity to devise a more sustainable and flexible strategy. Such a strategy must incorporate uncompromised patient care, a supportive clinical learning environment, direct academic and clinical teaching, relationship-building between academic and clinical staff, relationship development between clinical staff and students (support for clinicians to support the students), continuous feedback to students on their progress, learning by repetition, peer teaching and learning and collegiality with peers.

Transforming the Clinical Learning Environment

Transforming the clinical learning environment required analysis of two key qualities: the physical nature of the environment and the people, including clinical and academic staff, and students. These qualities reflected the partnering institutions' mission, vision, policy, finances and management structures.

The Physical Nature of the Environment

The DEU had to accommodate the variety of geographic locations (type and condition of buildings, space/ward layout, facilities and resources including staff and signage) and the clinical context (type of ward, type of care, number of patients, technology, rosters, tasks, routines and rituals).

The People

The calibre, attitudes and attributes of clinical staff in relation to their engagement with students and academic staff were of overwhelming significance in the clinical learning environment. Understanding their perceptions of their roles and responsibilities, their professional competence and their capacity to communicate effectively, role model, provide feedback and coach the students in patient care activities was paramount.

Similar to the impact of clinical staff, the calibre, attitudes and attributes of the academic staff were known to have an enormous influence on the clinical learning environment. Thus, it was necessary to understand academics' respect for, and collegiality with, each other, clinicians and students; their capacity to protect the students and patients; their perceptions of their role and responsibilities; their sense of responsibility to fulfil their role and responsibilities (e.g. being on the ward when they should be); and their capacity to communicate effectively, role model, provide feedback, coach the students in patient care activities, extend students' learning, assess students' progress and identify areas needing extra attention or for potential research.

The impact of students' attitudes and attributes on the dynamics of the relationships that developed during clinical placement had to be acknowledged. This encompassed their levels of respect for the clinical and academic staff and other students, their perceptions of themselves as learners and nurses, their willingness to take an active role in their learning, their maturity, readiness to take the risk of practising nursing and ability to function collegially and their communication skills.

Patients and other staff, while acknowledged as integral to the clinical learning environment, were not directly involved in the development of the DEU.

The Design

Designing the DEU as a sustainable clinical learning environment in a climate of reduced resources required identification of key characteristics that could best achieve sustainability: sustained relationships built on trust and respect; flexibility, depending on who is available and the working context (role-dependent rather than individual-dependent); adaptability to changing conditions whether these be personnel, finance, resources, management or policy changes in the university and/or the health service; recruitment and retention of clinical staff with the calibre of expertise needed to effectively facilitate students' clinical learning and the desire to work in the DEU environment; and better use of available resources.

Resource efficiency was achieved by placing more students in fewer venues for longer, thus reducing administration time and costs (SEE theory—'So Easy for Everyone') and building staff's educational and professional capacity through preparation, timely support and valuing their initiatives. Student learning outcomes, curriculum content, timetabling and overall costs also had to be factored in.

Having identified the characteristics of the DEU clinical learning environment design, my colleagues and I formulated a set of foundational guiding principles.

Clinicians and academics standing alongside each other and acknowledging each other's strengths—clinicians are expert practitioners; academics are expert educators

Relationships between the two built on mutual trust, respect and open communication

Clinicians and academics, through close relationships, creating a strong, collaborative, collegial partnership between the health service, clinical venue and university

Collaborative learning and teaching with academics, clinicians and students

Preparation—all involved know their roles, responsibilities and actions

Ongoing academic and clinical practice development of staff and students

We believed these would best drive an environment in which students received better preparation towards becoming graduate RNs; academics had greater opportunities to establish sustained relationships with clinical staff and students while maintaining their clinical skills and enhancing their teaching skills; and clinical staff had greater opportunities to establish sustained relationships with academics and students, understand the university nursing curriculum and enhance their clinical teaching skills.

Based on these principles, the DEU worked to everyone's advantage. All staff and students were valued as members of a care and teaching/learning team, seeking each other's feedback and using it to make improvements. Students had more opportunities to spend more time in clinical; to engage with intentional and incidental learning, including strategic and incidental peer teaching and learning; to learn through repetition; and to develop a sense of collegiality with their peers and practitioners.

Clinical staff were no longer disadvantaged. They, like academic staff, benefited from preparation for their teaching roles (including assessment) in the DEU before the students arrived and appreciation of, and reward for, their effort.

Establishing the Dedicated Education Unit

The primary step in establishing the DEU was negotiating with the School of Nursing to introduce and implement this innovation (see Chap. 4, this volume, for the story about implementation of the original DEU). Once this had been achieved, I, as Clinical Placement Coordinator (CPC), contacted the health service venue, and an institutional-level in-principle-agreement was established. The CPC approached individual heads of clinical units/wards (Clinical Nurse Consultants—CNCs) to set up DEUs. Part of the setting up process was developing new, clearly defined roles and their attendant responsibilities and actions so that whoever took a particular role knew the requirements. There was some crossover of actions for each role, as shown in Table 2.3.

Table 2.3 Actions for each key role in the DEU

Role	Actions
Principal Academic (PA)	Establish and maintain relationships to ensure student learning opportunities and objectives and to address issues inherent in DEU dynamics, by having conversations with individual academic staff, eliciting feedback about student progress and identifying initiatives recommended by staff for enhancing learning
A permanent School of Nursing lecturer responsible for liaising with the students, the Liaison Nurse (LN) and the CNC and utilising their ongoing expertise to facilitate students' learning	Maintain reliable and trustworthy communication between all parties
	Provide information about students to the clinical venue prior to students' arrival
	Hold meetings with the clinical staff outlining the nature of student learning objectives
	Participate with the CNC in selection of the LN, either per semester or yearly
	Collaborate with the LN to ensure initial rosters for students are configured and expectations re student behaviour are made clear (e.g. uniforms)
	Support orientation of students when they arrive in the DEU
	Facilitate student learning by overseeing their activities, questioning them about their patient care planning and implementation and challenging their transfer of theory into practice
	Initially role model patient care, including skills
	Support students in peer teaching roles
	Provide formative and summative evaluation of students both individually and in consultation with other clinical staff
	Continuously evaluate the DEU for its impact on the clinical venue and ability to meet students' learning objectives
	In conjunction with the CNC and LN, and dependent on their expectations and resources, encourage clinical staff to participate in the DEU by providing ideas and identifying issues, preferably before they become problems
	Identify potential for professional and research involvement
Clinical Nurse Consultant (CNC)	Communicate with the university and the hospital re having a DEU
Most senior nurse in the DEU responsible for overall running of the ward or clinical unit	Negotiate the capacity for a DEU within their unit—work out the organisational implications of having additional students
	Agree to have the DEU
	Advocate for students with the hospital management
	Ensure overall effectiveness of the DEU, alongside the PA

(continued)

Table 2.3 (continued)

Role	Actions
	Highlight the implications for the DEU dynamics (e.g. having so many people on the ward or unit)
	Identify and communicate to the university potential changes that might impact on students' learning (e.g. impending ward closure)
	Monitor and evaluate the impact of the DEU on staff and patients
	Maintain appropriate staffing levels
	Support staff to fulfil DEU objectives
	Support student learning (e.g. run seminars for the students in the clinical venue)
	Act as a role model and participate in students' clinical training and education
Liaison Nurse (LN)	Act as a conduit between PA and clinical staff
Full time RN responsible for overseeing clinical in the DEU	Communicate with the CNC re clinical in the DEU
	Keep clinical staff informed about what is happening with the DEU
	Keep the PA informed of any significant changes in the ward (e.g. policy changes)
	Organise orientation programmes for students on arrival in the DEU
	Manage roster changes
	Assess students—write final reports in consultation with the PA
	Fulfil their RN obligations in the ward but work with students alongside them, especially students who are having difficulties
	Be proactive in assessment of student problems
	Work with the PA to implement strategies to overcome problems
Clinicians	Initially demonstrate patient care
Registered nurses (RNs) and enrolled nurses (ENs) recognised for their expertise as clinician educators for students, responsible for facilitating students' learning in collaboration with the PA and LN	Over several shifts, evaluate students' preparedness for greater degrees of autonomy
	Provide students with timely and appropriate feedback
	Identify students' strengths and areas needing improvement
	Participate in weekly or fortnightly meetings with other staff, the PA and LN to review students' progress. Discuss different staff experiences with each individual student to identify where students are meeting objectives and where students need more input or focus
	Maintain communication with LN and PA
	Initiate other learning opportunities with students
	Suggest what else is available for the students
Clinical Placement Coordinator (CPC)	Negotiate clinical placements with clinical venues

(continued)

Table 2.3 (continued)

Role	Actions
Academic in the School of Nursing responsible for negotiating clinical placements, and ensuring placements were congruent with curriculum requirements for the whole undergraduate programme	Work out which venues can be used and when Supervise DEU clinical staff Work with the Clinical Placement Officer (general administrative staff in the School of Nursing) to ensure students have an appropriate variety of placements over the duration of their undergraduate programme (i.e. experience in acute medical surgical, operating room, accident and emergency, paediatrics and community placements such as drug and alcohol services) Resolve administrative or procedural issues in the clinical setting (bring in appropriate resources and people to resolve them if needed)
Clinical Placement Officer (CPO)	Work with the Clinical Placement Coordinator to ensure students have an appropriate variety of placements
General administrative staff member in the School of Nursing responsible for student placement and administration	Facilitate documentation of formal agreements/memorandums of understanding between the health services and the university re such things as legal issues Notify students of their placements Notify venues re student names and arrival schedules

Other factors considered for some of these roles included:

- Ideally, the PA had an opportunity to develop a DEU in their area of expertise, thus maintaining currency. Depending on the size of the DEU, the PA had approximately 10 h of student contact each week for the duration of the students' clinical learning placement (e.g. 14 weeks in the clinical setting, 1 week for preparation beforehand, and 1 week after for assessment and finalising the placement).
- The CNC, due to the nature of their role, was the primary initial contact in setting up the DEU.
- The PA and the CNC selected the LN, who was a clinical expert in their area. The LN was remunerated by up-classification from RN to clinical nurse (CN) in recognition of the responsibility of overseeing clinical in the DEU. The LN had four supernumerary days per semester (2 days for orientation and capacity building and 2 days for assessment at the end of semester) over and above their up-classification.
- Clinicians guided students initially from observation through to more autonomous practice, facilitating students' progression as learners and nurses. The clinicians became 'Clinician Educators' as students became more autonomous, a role that placed responsibility for learning on the student rather than on the clinician.

Student Learning Outcomes and Curriculum Content

The DEU design enhanced clinician and academic facilitation of student learning objectives and maintained the academic curriculum principle of achievable learning. More time for students in the clinical venues and more opportunities to practise combined with the collegiality of clinical and academic staff resulted in staff providing each other with information about individual students. This assisted staff to identify potential opportunities to enhance a student's learning for the best overall learning outcomes. Academics might identify additional learning objectives and dynamic interactions for the students and the clinical staff. Regular, ongoing and sustained contact between the clinicians and academics enabled early resolution of concerns and helped avert problems before they arose.

Timetabling

Timetable changes, creating minimal initial disruption to sequencing in the classroom, were offset by getting more students into appropriate learning venues. The most readily adaptable schedule was to have students in the clinical venues for 2 days per week, two shifts per day over 14 weeks. This timetabling was flexible in consideration of such things as numbers of students, numbers of clinical venues and curriculum changes. Trial and error was the ultimate determinant.

Cost

Some additional cost was envisaged in the set-up stage, but once the DEU was operational, its maintenance costs were less than for other clinical placement models. Savings of approximately 20 % per student in administration and clinical supervision costs were possible because there were more students per unit with only one PA and one LN on-site at all times, plus the RNs and ENs.

Implementing the Dedicated Education Unit

Implementation, management and the success of the DEU depended on collaboration among a critical mass of like-minded people in both the School of Nursing and the health services. This required dissemination of a draft DEU concept to the school discussion groups and the health services/hospitals with which the school had clinical placement arrangements. A joint meeting of these stakeholders was held to gain their feedback about the proposed DEU structure, the possibility of putting the DEU into action and, if they agreed to run with it, to form a steering committee to oversee its introduction. Implementation of DEUs in different contexts is detailed in Chaps. 4, 5, 6, 7, 8 and 11 in this volume.

Ownership

The principles provided a solid foundation on which to build a sense of collegial engagement and ownership; a sense developed through collective input by members of the school's current working groups and the creation of a DEU steering committee consisting of university and health services/hospital staff. Ongoing collaboration between university and health services/hospital staff strengthened the sense of ownership. Shared ideas, leadership, responsibility, action and ongoing feedback, as well as willingness to change in response to feedback, enhanced the sustainability of the DEU as a clinical teaching/learning strategy, an environment that was in tune with change and could flex accordingly.

What Did the DEU Look Like?

The DEU, dependent on strong, respectful relationships, communication and collaboration between health services and the university and among students, academics and clinical staff, was conceptualised as a hospital ward or health service unit in which Flinders University nursing students from all undergraduate year levels undertook placement. Placement was spread over a 14-week period from the beginning of Week 2 of semester until the end of Week 15 of semester. The number of students in the unit at any given time increased gradually as 2nd and then 1st year students joined the 3rd year students, for example:

- Week 1—preparation: preclinical meeting for the students with the PAs
- Week 2—10 × 3rd year students in clinical for 2 days per week for 12 weeks
- Week 6—10 × 2nd year students in clinical attached to the 3rd year students for 2 days per week for 10 weeks
- Week 10—6 × 1st year students in clinical attached to the 2nd year students for 2 days per week for 2 weeks
- Week 13—6 × 1st year students in clinical attached to the 2nd year students for 2 days per week for 2 weeks

The illustration at the beginning of the chapter (Fig. 2.1) emphasised the student-centredness of this configuration. The DEU was truly dedicated to optimal student learning.

Conclusion

Having conceptualised the DEU as a new clinical learning strategy in collaboration with my colleagues, I proceeded to canvass Flinders University School of Nursing staff and health service representatives in the southern area of Adelaide, South Australia, to trial it. Judy Gonda (Chap. 4, this volume) details the resultant trialling and implementation of Flinders University DEUs in health services in Adelaide, South Australia. Its uptake by other universities is described in Chap. 5 (University of Canberra, Australia), Chap. 6 (University of Portland, Oregon, North America), Chap. 7 (Christchurch Polytechnic Institute of Technology and Canterbury District Health Board [CPIT/CDHB], New Zealand) and Chap. 8 (University of Borås, Sweden), all in this volume.

Reference

Longson, D., Orrell, J., Edgecombe, K., & Gonda, J. (1997). Changes, challenges and chances in clinical teaching: transfer of learning between clinical practice and the University classroom. In Association of Practical Experiences in Professional Education (PEPE), *Proceedings, Third National Cross Faculty Practicum Conference*, Adelaide.

Chapter 3
The Dedicated Education Unit in Nursing as a Community of Practice

Laurie Grealish, Kasia Bail, and Jo Gibson

Glossary of Terms in Order of Appearance in This Chapter

Community of practice a community of people involved in mutual engagement (a network of multiple relationships between members of the community), having a shared repertoire ('routines, words, tools, ways of doing things, stories, gestures, symbols, genres, actions or concepts that the community has produced or adopted in the course of its existence') (Wenger 1998: 83) and collectively negotiating day-to-day practice (joint enterprise)

Preceptorship model one student allocated to one preceptor (an experienced RN who provides one-on-one support for nursing students)

Peer learning students learn with and from peers; students across different year levels learning together

Apprenticeship model old hospital-based model in which students learn from more senior clinical staff in the hospital

Principal Academic (PA) an academic lecturer in clinical (nursing school faculty member) who visits the clinical setting prior to student placement to

L. Grealish (✉)
Faculty of Health, University of Canberra, Canberra, ACT, Australia
e-mail: laurie.grealish@canberra.edu.au

K. Bail
Centre for Research and Action in Public Health, University of Canberra, Canberra, ACT, Australia
e-mail: Kasia.Bail@canberra.edu.au

J. Gibson
Canberra, ACT, Australia
e-mail: JGibson@anmac.org.au

K. Edgecombe and M. Bowden (eds.), *Clinical Learning and Teaching Innovations in Nursing*, Innovation and Change in Professional Education 10,
DOI 10.1007/978-94-007-7232-8_3,

facilitate clinical staff preparation for working with the students and thereafter visits the clinical setting regularly throughout each semester

Critical companionship a helping relationship in which an experienced facilitator accompanies another on an experiential learning journey, using methods of 'high challenge' and 'high support' in a trusting relationship (Titchen 2003)

Magnet Hospital a hospital that has been awarded recognition by the American Nurses Credentialing Center as a hospital that demonstrates excellence in nursing care

Introduction

Nursing in Australia, as in other developed countries, underwent significant changes in the latter part of the twentieth century. In an enormous undertaking, nursing education was moved from the health (hospital) sector into the higher education sector over a 10-year period from 1985 to 1994. The Dedicated Education Unit (DEU), a relatively new phenomenon in clinical education, arose in response to this change.

As with other courses in the university sector, it was assumed that learning about nursing was a cognitive activity and learning gained in the classroom could be applied to practice on graduation. Moving nursing students from a captive workforce into the world of learning (research) aimed to support the development of critical thinking about practice (Bolton 1981; Bottorff and D'Cruz 1985; Hart 1985; Watson 1982). Whilst nurse leaders at the time of the transfer valued higher education traditions, there were challenges to the assumption that learnt theory could be simply *applied* to practice for occupations such as nursing (Clare 1993).

The Transfer of Nursing Education into the University Sector

The transfer of nursing education into the higher education sector required new partnerships between higher education agencies and tertiary health services. Initially, higher education providers and health services formed exclusive partnerships that became unsustainable over time due to increased student numbers. New partnerships with services in the community (Bartz and Dean-Baar 2003) and aged care emerged to support student learning. They explored a range of student learning models, including:

- University-appointed clinical teachers working with groups of students—clinical supervision (Grealish and Carroll 1998; Kermode 1984)
- Health agency staff appointed as clinical teachers (Davies et al. 1999)
- An academic researcher appointed to the nursing team (Downie et al. 2001)

- Staff nurse preceptors for students in their final placement (Grealish and Carroll 1998)
- Peer learning (Aston and Molassiotis 2003; Lewis 1998)
- The Dedicated Education Unit (Edgecombe et al. 1999)

Early advocates for the transfer of nursing education argued for students to be supernumerary, rather than counted as a member of the team, so that they could be dedicated to learning whilst in the workplace (Watson 1982; Patten 1979). Despite general agreement that nursing students required learning opportunities in the workplace, the nature of that experience continued to be contested. Models for clinical education emphasised the need for nursing students to observe 'good' practice (role models) (Howie 1988; Kanitsaki and Sellick 1989) and openly examined the clinical workplace as a learning environment (Dunn and Hansford 1997; Hart and Rotem 1994).

By the turn of the century, nurse educators were arguing for immersion into nursing practice (Edmond 2001), suggesting that experience of nursing work increased critical thinking (Maynard 1996) and developed clinical scholarship (Elberson and Williams 1996). However, a devastating nursing shortage was emerging, and models of clinical learning favoured at the time of the transfer were proving problematic. Staff perceived students as a burden (Davey 2002), and students felt exploited as unpaid labour (Elliot 2002a). The exclusive relationships between higher education and health services were no longer satisfactory. Multiple relationships between the two sectors emerged, raising the need for explicit governance arrangements, such as contracts outlining the terms of specific relationships between organisations. Educational models that provided opportunities for students and staff to work together for longer periods were attractive for recruitment purposes, whereby students could 'try out' a particular workplace and managers could talk about future employment opportunities.

Learning in the clinical environment was the subject of research at the turn of the century, focusing on expert commentary in nursing specifically and in higher education more broadly. Some experts suggested that the workplace operated counter to a learning environment (Hughes 1998; Ward and McCormack 2000) because students, appreciating that the work experience placement is an opportunity to impress future employers, worked to hide their weaknesses. Thus, they avoided the challenges necessary to develop critical thinking and deep learning (Hughes 1998). Other authors describe this phenomenon as 'don't rock the boat' (Chapman and Orb 2001).

Teaching strategies to support learning shifted from the observational or limited participation models adopted initially in higher education programmes to a 'modified' apprenticeship in the form of preceptorship or mentorship (Morton-Cooper and Palmer 1993). In these two clinical learning models, the clinician was the primary source for learning, explaining her or his practice to the student. Such explanations are time-consuming for the clinician and can lead to their perception that students are a burden. The preceptorship model was not only demanding of the individual clinical preceptor, but there was emerging evidence that it continued to reproduce practice (Eraut 2004). It provided limited opportunity for students to question taken-for-granted assumptions and develop critical thinking skills (Andrews and Roberts 2003; Smith 2001). Whilst preceptorship is not supported in the DEU model, students will often identify mentors within the DEU team and work more closely with these nurses.

Facilitation of learning in the workplace by an 'outsider' can lead to deep learning (Hughes 1998). Facilitators, focusing on the learner's intent and developing learning strategies and activities appropriate to that intent (Boud and Walker 1990), can point out important things in what is a complex and murky clinical environment (Edgecombe and Bowden 2009; Papp et al. 2002). Facilitation is a foundational teaching strategy in the DEU model.

Peer learning is another foundational learning strategy in the DEU model. It is where students learn together in homogenous year groups (Lewis 1998) or where senior students work with junior students (Aston and Molassiotis 2003). Peer learning provides opportunities for students to develop their confidence around practice without observation by future employers or assessors. Whilst this approach is increasing in usefulness, the need for validation of learning through formative assessment is essential.

On the cusp of the twenty-first century, Dedicated Education Units emerged in Adelaide (Edgecombe et al. 1999), Clinical Development Units emerged in Sydney (Parsons and Mott 2003) and professorial units were introduced in Melbourne (Baker and Pearson 1991). In each of these models, the collaborative relationship between the health service staff and higher education staff is critical to student learning (Davies et al. 1999). The DEU model emerged in a time of change in nursing and nursing education, whereby initial assumptions about learning, based upon the academy's traditions, proved inadequate for nursing programmes and their graduates.

The Dedicated Education Unit Model

Edgecombe et al. (1999) suggest that the Dedicated Education Unit (DEU) model emerged for the pragmatic reasons outlined in Table 3.1, which Edgecombe discussed in Chap. 2 (this volume).

The impact of the transition of nursing education into the higher education sector is evident in these reasons. When the clinical environment is not structured to support student learning, staff express feelings of burden from having students from many different universities, and students do not have enough time in one practice setting to develop confidence in the practice and theory of nursing work. Research into the DEU model indicates benefits in the areas of student experience, service delivery, staff experience and partnership (Table 3.2). Whilst small sample sizes and qualitative design limit the generalisability of the findings, the evidence from each study in the table consistently reinforces the value of the DEU model for students, staff and the respective health and academic organisations. The personal stories shared in Chap. 10 (this volume) also reveal these benefits.

Table 3.1 Reasons for the DEU model (From Edgecombe et al. 1999)

Learning	Short condensed block placements do not give adequate opportunity for students to consolidate nursing skills performance, integrate theory and practice, promote understanding of the role and function of staff in clinical areas, allow for consolidation of *ANMC Competencies* and engender a sense of belonging
	Clinicians focus on task completion and may not facilitate theoretical integration
Teaching	Clinical staff expect to supervise and support student learning with little knowledge of their learning requirements
	Students express feeling that they receive insufficient assistance and guidance from academics
	Students report conflicting messages from classroom teachers and clinicians
Workload	Clinicians report feeling stressed by the student supervision role, and this may be exacerbated by short frequent student placements from a number of universities

Table 3.2 Research evidence related to the DEU

Students	Students value the weekly 2-day placement and associated opportunity to repeat practices to develop skills, experience different events, develop and consolidate knowledge and reflect on learning (Gonda et al. 1999)
	Students feel accepted and that they are making a contribution to the unit (Moscato et al. 2007; Ranse and Grealish 2007; Wotton and Gonda 2004)
	Students feel responsible for practice and that responsibility triggers learning (Grealish and Ranse 2009)
	Student relationships are fostered (Wotton and Gonda 2004)
Service delivery	Quality patient care is maintained (Wotton and Gonda 2004) and advanced (Mulready-Shick et al. 2009)
Staff	Clinical staff report greater opportunities for 'teachable moments' (Mulready-Shick et al. 2009)
	Clinical staff report valuing students for their 'fresh' eyes in residential aged care (Grealish et al. 2010)
	Clinical staff report feeling that they are making an investment in the future of the profession (Grealish et al. 2010)
Partnership	A greater sense of collaboration between clinicians, students and academics emerges (Wotton and Gonda 2004)

In a recent editorial, Tanner (2010) suggests that the DEU may provide a clinical education framework that can lead to the deep learning required for nursing practice. As noted earlier, during the transfer of nursing from the health sector to the higher education sector, there were calls for nursing students to be supernumerary and observers of practice—calls to stop the apprenticeship model dominant in hospital education. However, the evidence that has emerged in the last 30 years supports the inclusion of nursing students into health service delivery teams and the value of holding students responsible for practice in order to facilitate deep learning. Billett's framework for learning in the workplace (Billett et al. 2004) provides the theoretical structure necessary to correlate the research findings to date and develop a robust research agenda around learning in the DEU.

A Theoretical Framework: Learning in the Workplace

Billett et al. (2004) provide a framework for understanding learning in the workplace as reciprocal processes between the affordances of the workplace and the individual agencies of those people, including students, who participate in that work. In this framework, learning is viewed as a social as well as cognitive activity, influenced by micro-social processes that shape activities and actions and, therefore, learning. In the workplace, routine work practices can reinforce and refine existing knowledge, and new knowledge can be produced by engagement in new activities and interactions.

Billett (2001) uses the term 'the invitational quality of the learning environment' to describe the features of the environment that bring students into its business or work. Research work undertaken soon after the transfer of nursing education indicated clear characteristics of the workplace that influenced students' experiences of learning, including being welcomed by staff (Hart and Rotem 1994). Research tools to assess the workplace as a learning environment emerged soon after (Dunn and Hansford 1997; Papp et al. 2002). Situational factors and social negotiations influence the affordances offered by the workplace (Billett et al. 2004; Suchman 1996; Wenger 1998) but undergo constant transformation, rendering measurement at one point unreliable for the future. Repeated measures are required to monitor trends and new forms of evaluation of workplace learning environments.

The individual agency of the people participating in the work practices also plays a significant role in learning. Individuals' values, beliefs and sociocultural background mediate individual engagement in practice (Mak et al. 1998). Engagement in multiple social practices at any one time (Wenger 1998) means that individuals' engagement in each of these practices will not be consistent. A student can fully engage in one practice and not another (Billett et al. 2004). In summary, learners' identities, derived from personal and social histories unique to each individual, guide their agentic learning.

In the Billett et al. (2004: 238) framework, there is 'an interdependence between what is afforded individuals by social practice, and how they elect to engage with and construct what is afforded to them by the social practice'. This interdependence is multiple, situated and complex. The individual's level of engagement in practice and the purposes of that engagement mediate the learning derived from practice (Billett et al. 2004). Tensions can arise when workplaces cannot afford the types of practices (or learning) individuals desire or see as important to their personal development or promotion (Billett et al. 2004). This is frequently the case when placing nursing students in a residential aged care facility (Alabaster 2007).

The high value nursing students place on interpersonal relationships (Lee et al. 2002) suggests that negotiations are an important aspect of learning in the workplace. The Billett et al. (2004) framework of workplace affordances, student agency and negotiation of practice, and therefore learning, provides a conceptual tool for analysing the DEU model of clinical education's contribution to educational theory and practice.

Clinical Environment Design in the Dedicated Education Unit: Developing a Community of Practice

In the DEU, when the workplace is theoretically constructed as a community of practice, mutual engagement, shared repertoire and joint enterprise (Wenger 1998) serve as useful concepts to understand workplace affordances. This approach is quite different from traditional analyses of the clinical workplace as a learning environment. In traditional learning environment research frameworks, individual roles in the clinical environment are assumed to influence student learning. Nurses researching clinical environment design identify the nurse manager or charge nurse (Dunn and Burnett 1995; Elliot 2002b; Papp et al. 2002), the clinical teacher (Hart and Rotem 1994) and clinicians (Jackson and Mannix 2001) as key elements for student learning. A focus on individuals and their nature can be partially helpful, but in an environment where there is a shortage of nurses, a shift in focus from the individuals and roles to how nursing practices are negotiated may prove helpful in shaping clinical learning experiences (Manley and McCormack 2003).

Mutual engagement in the practices and actions of delivering care to patients, clients or residents of a health service implies membership of the community. Mutual engagement describes a network of multiple relationships between members of the community, some of which may be geographically located at a distance (Wenger 1998). Students must be mutually engaged in that community's practice in order to learn from clinical experience. Students are not only welcomed into the community but are allocated with challenging tasks suitable to their level of ability and afforded the opportunity to do these tasks with other members of the community.

The *shared repertoire* of a community of practice includes 'routines, words, tools, ways of doing things, stories, gestures, symbols, genres, actions or concepts that the community has produced or adopted in the course of its existence' (Wenger 1998: 83). Members create meaningful statements about their world, as well as their identities as members, from these repertoires. The inherently ambiguous nature of the repertoire of practice allows it to become a resource for negotiating meaning and therefore learning. Not only do students who are novices within the community learn from these negotiations, but there is potential for staff to learn as well (Grealish et al. 2010).

The third characteristic of a community of practice is the negotiation of a *joint enterprise*. Collective negotiations about practice involve members in mutually engaging in a complex network of relationships that define the community's joint enterprise (Wenger 1998). Rather than a mission statement or organisational goal, joint enterprise is situated and multiple; it is evident in the everyday practices of that community. It is the members' negotiated response to their situation and thus belongs to them in a profound sense—the community and individual identity is closely bounded through these day-to-day negotiations around practice. In an aged care facility, for example, joint enterprise is negotiated through giving medications, helping a resident with their meal, gently touching a relative's arm and singing a resident to sleep. Many people are involved in care delivery with many approaches to practice that require continuous negotiation and sometimes reification through procedural policy. Mutual accountability, which can be a great motivator for continued learning, is developed within the construct of joint enterprise (Wenger 1998).

Learner Agency: Learning and Identity in a Community of Practice

The emphasis on the learning environment is only part of the story of student learning. As Billett et al. (2004) and Boud and Prosser (2002) suggest, how students learn is fundamentally related to how they perceive their learning environment—how it is experienced rather than how it is designed. The idea of agency as a concept can contribute to our understanding of how students' perceptions influence learning.

The negotiation of practice, addressed in the previous section, is not necessarily something that is discussed within a community of practice. Negotiation does not require words, but words can be used. Members in a community of practice may not address negotiation directly, but it is revealed in the ways they engage in action with, and relate to, each other. These practices guide how to be a human being. Therefore, the formation of a community of practice is also the negotiation of identities (Wenger 1998). Glen (1998: 96) supports this theory, suggesting that 'individuals achieve by transcendent self-realisation through their relationships with other persons'.

Identity has a temporal dimension where it is continuously negotiated within the various communities to which an individual belongs (Wenger 1998). Whilst engaging in practice, an individual is simultaneously working with the situation at hand, participating in the histories (and possibly forming the futures) of certain practices and becoming, or transforming, identity. When identity is conceptualised as a trajectory, it provides a context within which to determine what is significant among the messy swamp of practice (Edgecombe and Bowden 2009); what becomes the focus of learning (Wenger 1998). This conceptualisation of identity is consistent with agency as defined by Billett et al. (2004), whereby the individual makes meaning, decides what is significant and, therefore, what is learnt, based on history and future goals. The individual perceives the world and, despite the 'best' learning environment as measured by contemporary instruments, may still not engage in the community's practice, thereby limiting opportunities to learn. It is paramount to design a curriculum to encourage individual participation as much as possible.

Teaching Practices and Assessment in the Dedicated Education Unit

Nursing is a practice-based discipline, and curriculum design inevitably must address the learning that occurs in the workplace. In an analysis of learning designs

Table 3.3 Four key areas for curriculum design (From Boud and Prosser 2002)

1. Engage learners from where they are, taking into account prior knowledge and intent
2. Acknowledge the learning context, the learner's context, the course of which the activity is part and the sites of application of the knowledge to be learnt
3. Challenge learners to be active participants, using other learners' support and stimulation, taking a critical approach to materials and to go beyond what is immediately provided
4. Provide practice where students demonstrate what is learnt, gain feedback and reflect on learning to develop confidence

for new technologies, Boud and Prosser (2002) outline four guidelines that would apply equally well in workplace learning design (Table 3.3).

Strategies *to engage learners from where they are* include finding out about them by asking questions about their backgrounds and using questions that reveal values, for example, 'What is most important in this situation for you?' Students can be encouraged to validate their conclusions with theory from their textbooks and the wisdom of more experienced nurses.

Recognising the reciprocal relationship between student agency and workplace affordances, strategies to *acknowledge the complexity of context* in clinical education might include:

- Prepare students for the learning context through information provision and a briefing or orientation session, being frank about what opportunities will not be available
- Support students to set learning goals that are consistent with what the placement experience can afford
- Recognise 'teachable moments' (Mulready-Shick et al. 2009) as they arise and use this to stimulate further learning
- Provide opportunities for students to repeat practices in different situations to develop confidence and recognise the influence of context
- Conduct workshops on negotiation theory and practice to support student participation in the clinical experience
- In debriefing or classroom activities, encourage students to share their experiences and think forward to other contexts in which this learning might apply

To *challenge students to be active participants*, teachers could:

- Provide a useful orientation to the nature of the work and values in that community of practice
- Encourage students to work in peer groups, across years as designed in the DEU, so that they can experience support from other students, and discuss what they are experiencing and learning with each other—reduce reliance on 'teachers'
- Avoid consistently explaining practice—let the students do the explaining, correct false conclusions and encourage further reading
- Ask comparative questions where the experience is compared to past experiences and possible future experiences
- Ask evaluative questions that require deep thought about value, quality and equity and require students to develop judgement

Finally, it is critical to students' development of confidence to provide them with opportunities *to demonstrate and receive feedback on what they have learnt* as practical, organisational or other skills and as knowledge. Whilst the *ANMC Competencies* (ANMC n.d.) provide a broad framework for giving feedback on performance, students also require specific feedback on authentic tasks or practices undertaken through participation (Elliot 2002b; Laurillard 1993).

Areas for Research

The DEU's theoretical underpinnings should be used as a guide to evaluation and research. We have identified four areas for research to stimulate thinking about possibilities in the development of the DEU model.

Curriculum design: Specifically, how learning and assessment are designed for integration into the overall programme is a key area for research. One of the core elements of the DEU is the extended placement in one area, visiting 2 or 3 days each week.

Pedagogies: These inform curriculum design, facilitate student learning, contribute directly to the invitational quality of the workplace and include assessment and feedback on learning.

Stakeholder engagement: This is foundational to the model, curriculum design and pedagogies. Ways of working with the increasing numbers of identified stakeholders in the DEU model are becoming increasingly important.

The DEU as a learning organisation: It shifts the focus from student learning to the organisation, and how working within a DEU model can improve organisational services and products.

Curriculum Design

The challenge of integrating learning from the workplace into the overall curriculum design is not unique to the DEU model. However, as the demand for clinical placements continues to rise, health agencies may seek to manage the workload associated with student placements through intensive or block, rather than extended placements. Further, some students prefer block placements for personal reasons. Universities are encouraged to support the increasing diversity of students as well as work with multiple placement partners, and, as such, curriculum design should integrate learning from both styles of placements.

Research into curriculum design could focus questions on the alignment of graduate outcomes, learning experiences and assessment practices using Biggs' (1999) concept of constructive alignment. Constructive alignment focuses on aligning the learning experiences (tasks, assessment, activities) with the intended learning outcomes. The focus is on how students piece together (construct) their learning. Consistency of learning activities towards the stated goals is important. Variables of block or extended placements for learning experiences could be tested in relation to student learning to determine whether there are significant benefits in either model.

In the Billett et al. (2004) framework, students are agentic learners and seek value in their learning; they make meaning based on their history and future goals. Therefore, curriculum design enables exposing students to experiences requiring negotiation and, as a result, meaning making or learning. The effectiveness of methods to facilitate negotiation and meaning making required in the clinical setting is worthy of further investigation.

The area of clinical assessment remains a challenging component of nursing education for clinicians and academics (Cowan et al. 2005; McAllister 1998). Further exploration would be valuable into how feedback on performance is practised best in accordance with the *ANMC Competencies* (ANMC n.d.) and on authentic tasks or practices undertaken through participation.

Pedagogies

A number of pedagogies can be seen to underlie the DEU. Further exploration of whether the high support, high challenge (Johns 1994) DEU environment can be seen to increase the reflective practice (Schön 1983; van Manen 1977) of students who experience it could be beneficial. Recent university emphasis on Graduate Attributes as an underpinning component of teaching philosophy may be clearly displayed in the DEU model and offer scope for evaluation (Barrie et al. 2009). Formative and summative assessment in the DEU (Biggs and Tang 2007), with a large emphasis on self-assessment, could be examined in comparison to other models. There is also increased scope in the DEU for 'ongoing summative assessments' because students are encouraged to plan their learning objectives for each component of their degree from year to year (not just subject to subject), based on their knowledge, experience and learning needs. Boud (2000) refers to 'sustained assessment' that fosters lifelong learning, which is well aligned with the DEU principles. This link offers an avenue to explore whether his theory applies to the DEU model.

One of the key pedagogies in the DEU is the use of peer learning, where students across year groups work together in the same clinical setting. Often, the 3rd year students are given the opportunity to lead in these environments. As Aston and Molassiotis (2003) note, when 3rd and 1st year students work and learn together, the 3rd year students require some preparation (pedagogies). The DEU model provides the opportunity for further investigation of student learning with peers and the phenomenon Billett et al. (2004) label 'interdependence'—how students in the workplace affect staff and student learning.

The role of the Principal Academic (PA) offers a wealth of information as to how pedagogy is applied in a clinical setting. Principles and theory on moderation of marking (Krieg et al. 2004), assessment (Biggs and Tang 2007) and even deep versus surface learning (Biggs 1999) are challenged when taken out of the academic context. Clinical support roles such as 'critical companionship' (Titchen 2003) may offer fruitful avenues of exploration. The ongoing tension between a student-focused 'critical companion' approach to academics' clinical engagement with students and the role of assessor is also worthy of investigation. Research into how nursing practices are negotiated may prove helpful for planning and evaluating clinical learning experiences (Manley and McCormack 2003).

Using the Billett et al. (2004) framework as a conceptual tool for analysing the DEU model of clinical education's contribution to educational theory and practice in different locations across the world would offer insight into what components of the DEU might consistently support the framework.

Stakeholder Engagement

In clinical education, there is a range of stakeholders (Lockwood 2003). Often, stakeholders can be grouped into 'industry' or 'employers', with little appreciation of the diversity of individuals in that group. For example, agency managers and senior university staff made the decision to establish and implement a new DEU in one tertiary level ward. The clinicians in this ward were not consulted in the process, and as a result the DEU was reported to be unsuccessful (Grealish and Kaye 2004). Research into stakeholder engagement must clearly identify the range of stakeholders involved in clinical education. Table 3.4 contains a beginning list.

The management of a range of relationships between universities and health agencies is a rich area for research. Relationship management is under-researched generally, and there is almost no research into the work of providing clinical learning experiences. The need for a governance or reference group in establishing the DEU is acknowledged (Owen and Grealish 2006) for ensuring a smooth transition and addressing issues and incidents as they emerge. However, many relationships exist between a range of stakeholders outside the governance group, producing a rich network which, to date, has not been mapped. Another area for research is the management of these networks and relationships, their subsequent impact on student learning and other possible relationships such as clinical research.

An expanding phenomenon is the use of clinical placement management systems. What would be the effect on established relationships of implementing computer programmes? How would it affect negotiation strategies? What would be the effect on student learning, patient care, clinician satisfaction and administrative workload? Thus, the implementation of computer programmes offers an interesting area of research.

Table 3.4 Potential stakeholders in clinical nursing education

University	Health agency	Other
Students	Chief executive officer	Chief nurse
Academic staff	Director of nursing	Professional associations
Sessional staff	Clinical nurses	Regulatory authorities
Administrative staff	Other clinicians	Alumni
Vice-chancellor	Patients/clients/residents	Specialist nurses
Head of nursing dept.	Families	Other education providers
	Unit manager	

The Dedicated Education Unit as a Learning Organisation

Whilst there is an agreement that learning experiences in the clinical environment are critical to nursing education, research to date has been constrained by limiting the conceptualisation of the clinical workplace as a learning environment to its people and surroundings. The development of the Clinical Learning Environment Scale (Dunn and Burnett 1995) and subsequent adoption of the 'clinical learning environment' as a researchable concept (Dunn and Hansford 1997) have led to significant levels of research in this area (see Chan 2002; Elliot 2002a; Papp et al. 2002; Saarikoski and Leino-Kilpi 2002). There has been limited commentary or research on the relationship between student learning and organisational learning. In one small qualitative study, Grealish et al. (2010) investigated the effects of having students in the residential aged care workplace and found that the presence of students encouraged staff learning as well. This falls short of the need for investigations into the role that the DEU could play in the learning organisation.

Organisational perspectives about the value of learning environments for nurses and patients, including the Magnet Hospital movement in the USA (Ulrich et al. 2007), could offer insight into how the DEU pedagogy aligns with preferred hospital providers' structure and function. Considering that the workplace as a learning organisation has developed traction in the discipline of management, Edmondson and Moingeon (1998) suggest that organisational viability in an environment characterised by uncertainty and change depends on individual and collective learning.

Learning organisations are those in which people continually expand their capacity to create the results they truly desire (Senge 2006). The presence of supportive values and beliefs that encourage employee inquisitiveness and creativity, a willingness to learn from error and openness to sharing knowledge are viewed as significant contributors to a learning organisation culture (Lee-Kelley et al. 2007). These qualities, noted in every instance of the recognisable learning organisation, are also valued in a clinical learning environment. Senge (2006) reinforces this view in relation to aspects of individual and team learning in organisations, referring to the fact that individuals learn all the time, yet there is no organisational learning. However, as teams learn, they become a 'microcosm for learning throughout the organisation' (Senge 2006: 219).

There is an emerging body of management literature describing interwoven workplace learning, employee engagement, organisational performance and broader economic, regulatory and social contexts within which organisations operate (Unwin et al. 2007). Unwin et al. (2007) point out that workplaces often have an advantage over 'formal' *educational* institutions in that pedagogic activity is likely to be spread across a broader range of people. Indeed, workplaces that recognise the pedagogic potential of their employees (and arguably hosted 'learners' in the context of the clinical environment) afford a stronger learning environment than those that conceptualise transmission of skills and knowledge as solely a top-down hierarchical approach (Smith and Billett 2006; Unwin et al. 2007). Investigations of student learning, within the broader context of learning organisations and management theories, may provide new and unique insights into the value of the DEU for health service agencies and universities.

Conclusion

This chapter set out to establish the underpinnings of the relatively new DEU clinical learning model by providing an overview of the history of clinical nursing education and research. Understanding the DEU as a community of practice and the value of social theories of learning for reconceptualising the workplace as a learning environment provides opportunities for further development of the DEU model. The consideration of literature beyond that of nursing education, including management literature on the learning organisation, is necessary to advance clinical nursing education theory and practice.

References

Alabaster, E. (2007). Involving students in the challenges of caring for older people. *Nursing Older People, 19*(6), 23–28.

Andrews, M., & Roberts, D. (2003). Supporting student nurses learning in and through clinical practice: The role of the clinical guide. *Nurse Education Today, 23*(7), 474–481.

ANMC (n.d.). *ANMC competencies*. Australian Nursing and Midwifery Council. http://www.nursingmidwiferyboard.gov.au/Codes-Guidelines-Statements/Codes-Guidelines.aspx. Accessed 16 Aug 2012.

Aston, A., & Molassiotis, A. (2003). Supervising and supporting student nurses in clinical placements: The peer support initiative. *Nurse Education Today, 23*(3), 202–210.

Baker, H., & Pearson, A. (1991). The experience of patients in a professorial nursing unit. *Australian Journal of Advanced Nursing, 9*(1), 15–19.

Barrie, S., Hughes, C., & Smith, C. (2009). *The national graduate attributes project: Integration and assessment of graduate attributes in curriculum*. Sydney: The Australian Learning and Teaching Council, University of Sydney.

Bartz, C., & Dean-Baar, S. (2003). Reshaping clinical nursing education: An academic-service partnership. *Journal of Professional Nursing, 19*(4), 216–222.

Biggs, J. (1999). *Aligning teaching for constructing learning*. York: Higher Education Academy. http://www.heacademy.ac.uk. Accessed 13 Feb 2010.

Biggs, J., & Tang, C. (2007). Aligning assessment tasks with intended learning outcomes: Principles. In Society for Research into Higher Education (Ed.), *Teaching for quality learning at university* (3rd ed., pp. 163–194). Buckingham: Society for Research into Higher Education.

Billett, S. (2001). Learning through work: Workplace affordances and individual engagement. *Journal of Workplace Learning, 13*(5), 209–214.

Billett, S., Barker, M., & Hernon-Tinning, B. (2004). Participatory practices at work. *Pedagogy, Culture and Society, 12*(2), 233–257.

Bolton, G. (1981). A training in discipline and conformity? *The Australian Nurses' Journal, 11*(4), 34–36.

Bottorff, J. L., & D'Cruz, J. V. (1985). The nursing curriculum and knowledge of most worth. *Australian Journal of Advanced Nursing, 2*(3), 9–17.

Boud, D. (2000). Sustainable assessment: Rethinking assessment for the learning society. *Studies in Continuing Education, 22*(2), 151–167.

Boud, D., & Prosser, M. (2002). Appraising new technologies for learning: A framework for development. *Education Media International, 39*(1), 237–245.

Boud, D., & Walker, D. (1990). Making the most of experience. *Studies in Continuing Education, 12*(2), 61–80.

Chan, D. (2002). The development of the Clinical Learning Environment Inventory: Using the framework of clinical learning environment studies to assess students' perceptions of the hospital as a learning environment. *Journal of Nursing Education, 41*(2), 69–75.

Chapman, R., & Orb, A. (2001). Coping strategies in clinical practice: The nursing students' lived experience. *Contemporary Nurse, 11*, 95–102.

Clare, J. (1993). Change the curriculum or transform conditions of practice? *Nurse Education Today, 13*(4), 282–286.

Cowan, D., Norman, I., & Coopamah, V. (2005). Competence in nursing practice: A controversial concept—A focused review of literature. *Nurse Education Today, 25*(5), 355–362.

Davey, L. (2002). Nurses eating nurses: The caring profession which fails to nurture its own. *Contemporary Nurse, 13*(2–3), 192–197.

Davies, E., Turner, C., & Osborne, Y. (1999). Evaluating a clinical partnership model for undergraduate nursing students. *Collegian, 6*(2), 23–27, 40.

Downie, J., Orb, A., Wynaden, D., McGowan, S., Zeeman, Z., & Ogilvie, S. (2001). A practice-research model for collaborative partnership. *Collegian, 8*(4), 27–32.

Dunn, S. V., & Burnett, P. (1995). The development of a clinical learning environment scale. *Journal of Advanced Nursing, 22*, 1166–1173.

Dunn, S. V., & Hansford, M. (1997). Undergraduate nursing students' perceptions of their clinical learning environment. *Journal of Advanced Nursing, 25*(6), 1299–1306.

Edgecombe, K., & Bowden, M. (2009). The ongoing search for best practice in clinical teaching and learning: A model of nursing students' evolution to proficient novice registered nurses. *Nurse Education in Practice, 9*(2), 91–101.

Edgecombe, K., Wotton, K., Gonda, J., & Mason, P. (1999). Dedicated Education Units 1: A new concept for clinical teaching and learning. *Contemporary Nurse, 8*(4), 166–171.

Edmond, C. B. (2001). A new paradigm for practice education. *Nurse Education Today, 21*(4), 251–259.

Edmondson, A., & Moingeon, B. (1998). From organizational learning to the learning organization. *Management Learning, 29*, 5–20.

Elberson, K., & Williams, S. (1996). Innovative strategies for promoting nursing scholarship: A holistic approach. *Holistic Nursing Practice, 10*(3), 33–40.

Elliot, M. (2002a). The Clinical Environment: A source of stress for undergraduate nurses. *Australian Journal of Advanced Nursing, 20*(1), 34–38.

Elliot, M. (2002b). Clinical education: A challenging component of undergraduate nursing education. *Contemporary Nurse, 12*(1), 69–77.

Eraut, M. (2004). Informal learning in the workplace. *Studies in Continuing Education, 26*(2), 247–273.

Glen, S. (1998). The key to quality nursing care: Towards a model of personal and professional development. *Nursing Ethics, 5*(2), 95–102.

Gonda, J., Wotton, K., Edgecombe, K., & Mason, P. (1999). Dedicated Education Units 2: An evaluation. *Contemporary Nurse, 8*(4), 172–176.

Grealish, L., & Carroll, G. (1998). Beyond preceptorship and supervision: A third clinical teaching model emerges for Australian nursing education. *Australian Journal of Advanced Nursing, 15*(2), 3–11.

Grealish, L., & Kaye, L. (2004). Change and challenge: The implementation of a new model of clinical learning for undergraduate nursing students in a cancer setting. *Australian Journal of Cancer Nursing, 5*(2), 3–4, 6–7, 9–11.

Grealish, L., & Ranse, K. (2009). An exploratory study of first year nursing students' experience of learning in the workplace. *Contemporary Nurse, 33*(1), 80–92.

Grealish, L., Bail, K., & Ranse, K. (2010). Investing in the future: Residential aged care staff experience of working with nurses in a 'community of practice'. *Journal of Clinical Nursing, 19*(15–16), 2291–2299. doi:10.1111/j.1365-2702.2009.03133.x.

Hart, G. (1985). College-based education: Background and bugs. *The Australian Nurses' Journal, 15*(4), 46–48.

Hart, G., & Rotem, A. (1994). The best and worst: Students' experience of clinical education. *Australian Journal of Advanced Nursing, 11*(3), 26–33.

Howie, J. (1988). The effective clinical teacher: A role model. *Australian Journal of Advanced Nursing, 5*(2), 23–26.

Hughes, C. (1998). Practicum learning: Perils of the authentic workplace. *Higher Education Research and Development, 17*(2), 207–227.

Jackson, D., & Mannix, J. (2001). Clinical nurses as teachers: Insights from students of nursing in their first semester of study. *Journal of Clinical Nursing, 10*, 270–277.

Johns, C. (1994). Guided reflection. In A. Palmer et al. (Eds.), *Reflective practice in nursing; The growth of the professional practitioner*. Oxford: Blackwell.

Kanitsaki, O., & Sellick, K. (1989). Clinical nurse teaching: An investigation of student perceptions of clinical nurse teacher behaviours. *Australian Journal of Advanced Nursing, 6*(4), 18–24.

Kermode, S. (1984). The role of the clinical supervisor in college programs. *The Australian Nurses' Journal, 13*(6), 34–35.

Krieg, S., Sharp, S., & Campbell, A. (2004, February 9–10). *Blurring the boundaries between teaching, learning, and assessment in a social constructivist framework: The use of rubrics as an educative tool.* In Seeking Educational Excellence. Proceedings of the 13th Annual Teaching Learning Forum, Murdoch University, Perth. http://lsn.curtin.edu.au/tlf/tlf2004/krieg.html. Accessed 10 July 2010.

Laurillard, D. (1993). *Rethinking university teaching: A framework for the effective use of educational technology*. London: Routledge.

Lee, W., Cholowski, K., & Williams, A. (2002). Nursing students' and clinical educators' perceptions of characteristics of effective clinical educators in an Australian university school of nursing. *Journal of Advanced Nursing, 39*(5), 412–420.

Lee-Kelley, L., Blackman, D., & Hurst, J. (2007). An exploration of the relationship between learning organizations and the retention of knowledge workers. *The Learning Organization, 14*(3), 204–221.

Lewis, M. (1998). An examination of the role of learning environments in the construction of nursing identity. *Nurse Education Today, 18*(3), 221–225.

Lockwood, C. (2003). *The effectiveness of undergraduate clinical placement, models, methods and meaningfulness for key stakeholders in South Australia* (pp. 1–38). Adelaide: Centre for Evidence based Nursing South Australia, The Joanna Briggs Institute.
Mak, A., Westwood, M. J., Barker, M. C., & Ishiyama, F. (1998). The ExceLL program for developing international students' sociocultural competencies. *Journal of International Education, 9*(1), 33–38.
Manley, K., & McCormack, B. (2003). Practice development: Purpose, methodology, facilitation and evaluation. *Nursing in Critical Care, 8*(1), 22–29.
Maynard, C. A. (1996). Relationship of critical thinking ability to professional nurse competence. *Journal of Nursing Education, 35*(1), 12–18.
McAllister, M. (1998). Competency standards: Clarifying the issues. *Contemporary Nurse, 7*(3), 131–137.
Morton-Cooper, A., & Palmer, A. (1993). *Mentoring and preceptorship: A guide to support roles in clinical practice*. Oxford: Blackwell.
Moscato, S. R., Miller, J., Logsdon, K., Weinberg, S., & Chorpenning, L. (2007). Dedicated Education Unit: An innovative clinical partner education model. *Nursing Outlook, 55*, 31–37.
Mulready-Shick, J., Kafel, K., Banister, G., & Mylott, L. (2009). Enhancing quality and safety competency development at the unit level: An initial evaluation of student learning and clinical teaching on Dedicated Education Units. *Journal of Nursing Education, 48*(12), 716–719.
Owen, J., & Grealish, L. (2006). Clinical education delivery. A collaborative, shared governance model provides a framework for planning, implementation and evaluation. *Collegian, 13*(2), 15–21.
Papp, I., Markkanen, M., & von Bonsdorff, M. (2002). Clinical environment as a learning environment: Student nurses' perceptions concerning clinical learning experiences. *Nurse Education Today, 23*, 262–268.
Parsons, M., & Mott, S. (2003). Royal Rehabilitation Centre Sydney: Towards clinical development units (nursing). *Collegian, 10*(1), 27–29.
Patten, M. (1979). College-trained for primary care. *The Australian Nurses Journal, 9*(2), 36–38, 52.
Ranse, K., & Grealish, L. (2007). Nursing students' perceptions of learning in the clinical setting of a Dedicated Education Unit. *Journal of Advanced Nursing, 58*(2), 171–179.
Saarikoski, M., & Leino-Kilpi, H. (2002). The clinical learning environment and supervision by staff nurses: Developing the instrument. *International Journal of Nursing Studies, 39*(3), 259–267.
Schön, D. (1983). *The reflective practitioner: How professionals think in action*. New York: Basic Books.
Senge, P. (2006). *The fifth discipline: The art and practice of the learning organization* (2nd ed.). London: Random House.
Smith, A. (2001). Nursing in a time of change: A case for critical thinking. *Contemporary Nurse, 19*, 194–200.
Smith, R., & Billett, S. (2006). Interdependencies at work: Reflection, performance, dialogue and reward. *Journal of Adult and Continuing Education, 12*(2), 156–169.
Suchman, L. (1996). Constituting shared workspaces. In Y. Engestrom & D. Middleton (Eds.), *Cognition and communication at work* (pp. 35–60). Cambridge: Cambridge University Press.
Tanner, C. (2010). From Mother Duck to Mother Lode: Clinical education for deep learning. *Journal of Nursing Education, 49*(1), 3–4.
Titchen, A. (2003). Critical companionship: Part 1. *Nursing Standard, 18*(9), 33–40.
Ulrich, B. T., Buerhaus, P. I., Donelan, K., Norman, L., & Dittus, R. (2007). Magnet status and registered nurse views of the work environment and nursing as a career. *Journal of Nursing Administration, 37*, 212–220.
Unwin, L., Felsted, A., Fuller, A., Bishop, D., Lee, T., Jewson, N., & Butler, P. (2007). Looking inside the Russian doll: The interconnections between context, learning and pedagogy in the workplace. *Pedagogy, Culture and Society, 15*(3), 333–348.
Van Manen, M. (1977). Linking ways of knowing to ways of being practical. *Curriculum Inquiry, 6*(3), 203–228.

Ward, C., & McCormack, B. (2000). Creating an adult learning culture through practice development. *Nurse Education Today, 20*, 259–266.

Watson, J. (1982). Traditional v. tertiary: Ideological shifts in nursing education. *The Australian Nurses' Journal, 12*(2), 44–46, 64.

Wenger, E. (1998). *Communities of practice: Learning, meaning and identity*. Cambridge: Cambridge University Press.

Wotton, K., & Gonda, J. (2004). Clinician and student evaluation of a collaborative clinical teaching model. *Nurse Education in Practice, 4*(2), 120–127.

Chapter 4
An 'Idea Whose Time Had Come': The Flinders University School of Nursing Dedicated Education Unit—An Historical Perspective

Judith (Judy) Gonda

Glossary of Terms in Order of Appearance in This Chapter

Nurse clinicians clinical staff

Nurse academics academic staff

Hospital-based apprenticeship model students learn from more senior clinical staff in the hospital and from each other

Supervision model traditional placement with an academic playing a supervisory role

Mentorship model one experienced registered nurse (RN) mentors a 3rd year student

Preceptorship model one student allocated to one preceptor (experienced RN)

Director of Nursing (DON) a registered nurse (RN) who supervises a whole nursing department

Clinical Nurse Consultant (CNC) most senior nurse in the DEU responsible for overall running of the unit

Registered Nurse (RN) college or university qualified nurse licensed by a nursing registration body to undertake all facets of nursing in accordance with the body's regulations

Enrolled Nurse (EN) diploma qualified nurse working under supervision of a RN to provide nursing care

J. (Judy) Gonda (✉)
Faculty of Health Sciences, Australian Catholic University, Brisbane, QLD, Australia
e-mail: Judith.Gonda@acu.edu.au

K. Edgecombe and M. Bowden (eds.), *Clinical Learning and Teaching Innovations in Nursing*, Innovation and Change in Professional Education 10,
DOI 10.1007/978-94-007-7232-8_4,

Principal Academic (PA) an academic lecturer in clinical (nursing school faculty member) who visits the clinical setting prior to student placement to facilitate clinical staff preparation for working with the students and thereafter visits the clinical setting regularly throughout each semester; communicates and liaises with students, the LN and the CNC, and utilises their ongoing expertise to facilitate students' learning

Liaison Nurse (LN) full-time registered nurse (RN) responsible for overseeing clinical in the DEU

Clinical Nurse (CN) a registered nurse (RN) accorded a position of seniority and experience

ANMC Competencies Australian Nursing and Midwifery Council competencies required for registration as a nurse (RN) and/or midwife (RM) (ANMC n.d.)

Introduction

In the late 1990s, clinical education for nurses faced a crisis. There was a dire need for a new perspective on how the profession should implement clinical education. It was also clear that whatever forms this took, there had to be a sense of joint ownership by nurse clinicians and nurse academics.

It was from within this context that Kay Edgecombe, a lecturer from the School of Nursing at Flinders University in South Australia, conceptualised the idea for the Dedicated Education Unit (DEU). The School faced the same issues as all other Schools of Nursing at that time—increasing student numbers, decreasing access to quality clinical learning environments for students and shrinking numbers of academics. In essence, the concept was simple. The DEU incorporated the best aspects of the original hospital-based apprenticeship model and of the supervision, mentorship and preceptorship models that followed (see Edgecombe, Chap. 2, this volume), and it was designed to use existing health care units more efficiently and creatively.

Once Kay had conceptualised the DEU in collaboration with nurse and academic colleagues, as described in Chap. 2 (this volume), she presented a rough draft to the School's academic discussion group. The group asked her to present it to a seminar with the Directors of Nursing (DON) from the Southern Health Care Providers who were placement partners with Flinders University. The placement partners fully supported the new concept, so Kay sought to test it by implementing a pilot DEU. This required assistance from others and the choice of who would do this was quite serendipitous. Kay approached the topic coordinators of clinical units from each year group of the Bachelor of Nursing for the following semester, who turned out to be Karen Wotton and me, as well as Kay. Whilst this was serendipitous, it was also pragmatic because Kay was aware that Karen and I were very passionate and concerned about the state of clinical education at that time.

Late in 1996, the three of us approached Peter Mason, the Clinical Nurse Consultant (CNC) of ward 5G at Flinders Medical Centre, to see if he would be interested in trialling this new clinical education model on that ward. We made this choice because:

- We felt it was imperative that we pilot the model in a conducive environment before we presented it with challenges.
- Kay and I had previously been clinical facilitators for groups of our students on ward 5G and had found it to be an excellent learning environment.
- It was apparent that Peter was committed to quality nursing education.

Consequently, we believed ward 5G was the best option. Fortunately, Peter was very enthusiastic (testimony to this is Story 7, Chap. 10, this volume).

As is evident from descriptions in the Introduction and Chaps. 2 (Edgecombe) and 3 (Grealish et al.) in this volume, the DEU concept embraces the philosophy of partnerships and incorporates the essential criteria required for their success. These criteria, identified by Mattessich and Monsey (1998), include six categories:

1. Purpose of the partnership
2. Environment
3. Structure and processes
4. Membership characteristics
5. Communication
6. Resources

For the remainder of this chapter, I describe the phases of the Flinders University DEU pilot implementation and use the above criteria to provide a framework throughout.

The Flinders University Dedicated Education Unit Pilot Implementation Phase 1

The first pilot DEU was implemented in Semester 1 of 1997. However, before the implementation of the pilot could occur, a proposal, justifying the pilot, was submitted to the 5th Floor Assistant Director of Nursing and the Ward Manager for 5G at Flinders Medical Centre, Adelaide, South Australia. This group approved the pilot study on 5G. From then on, implementation issues were primarily decided in collaboration between Kay, Karen, Peter and I, referred to as *the implementation team*.

Purpose

For some time in the mid-1990s, academics, clinicians and students in South Australia had expressed dissatisfaction with the models of clinical placement implemented by the tertiary Schools of Nursing during that time. Reasons for this dissatisfaction arose from:

- Inadequate time spent by students in the clinical area
- Inadequate time for students to repeatedly practise clinical skills
- Students' inability to transfer classroom learning into practice
- Lack of collaboration between academia and clinicians
- Students' difficulties in the transition to the registered nurse (RN) role
- Clinicians' frustration as a result of multiple groups of students with differing goals and expectations

Consequently, the purpose of the DEU pilot was to implement and evaluate a clinical placement model that could overcome these problems. In addition, it was expected that outcomes from evaluation of the pilot would indicate that:

1. Nursing students were more appropriately prepared for clinical practice by participating in the DEU.
2. There was greater integration of the academics and clinicians from each participating organisation as a result of the DEU.
3. Nursing clinicians would experience greater satisfaction in their role as student facilitators as a consequence of this model.
4. Relationships between practice-based nursing and the academic discipline were enhanced as a result of the DEU.

Environment

Flinders Medical Centre is a relatively new (opened in 1976) secondary level public hospital. Its principal operational areas are the care of acutely ill patients (adults and children), obstetric care, medical research and the education of medical and allied health care workers. It has always been closely associated with Flinders University as it was included in the original University plans and therefore was an obvious choice for the first pilot DEU.

During the second half of 1997, the hospital offered approximately 500 acute care and obstetric beds to the community in the Southern area of Adelaide. Ward 5G was a highly acute, 28-bed unit, specialising in the care of patients experiencing gastro-intestinal and hepato-biliary medical and surgical problems. It was also the liver transplant unit for South Australia and the Northern Territory and had a small number of beds for patients requiring eye surgery.

The unit was well resourced with the most up-to-date equipment. Medical and nursing interventions were evidence-based and cutting edge. There was also a multitude of students from a variety of health care disciplines, such as medicine, physiotherapy, occupational therapy and nutrition. Consequently, plenty of learning opportunities from a diversity of disciplinary, theoretical and practical perspectives were available for nursing students.

At that time, it could be said that the ward was not well staffed number-wise, but what it lacked in numbers it made up for in experience.

Structure and Process

Clinician Preparation

Before anything could proceed with the pilot study, we wanted to ensure that the majority of the RNs and enrolled nurses (ENs) on the ward were informed about the project and conducive to participating.

In the first instance, Peter met with senior staff from the ward and put the idea to them. As there was already a culture of education in the unit, it wasn't hard to convince them and they were keen to participate. However, they had some reservations, particularly about the high student numbers and the peer teaching/learning.

Subsequently, we held a series of informal staff meetings during the shift change-over time, a time of double staff numbers. We invited as many of the nurses who could attend to each meeting where we provided an overview of what the DEU was and the purpose behind it. The aim was to inform as many nurses as possible about the pilot project. We described how the DEU would be operationalised and then clarified different aspects of it. However, these meetings primarily provided an opportunity for the clinical staff to voice their concerns—to be heard—and for us to mutually work out ways to overcome potential problems and allay their fears.

In addition to these meetings, a 1-day workshop was provided on the University campus for ward staff who could be released from clinical duties for the day. This workshop included a brief overview of the DEU concept, an introduction to teaching/learning theory and some clinical teaching strategies.

Student Recruitment and Preparation

It was decided that in this first pilot, the DEU would accommodate 14 3rd year, 14 2nd year and 8 1st year students, a total of 36 students. The students were recruited by asking them to submit a written expression of interest to participate. However, as the clinical hours in the DEU would be greater than that expected of other students in the course, they were advised to take into account financial/paid work requirements and family commitments before applying.

A short meeting was held with potential participants to provide an overview of the DEU concept and to inform them of the shift requirements and start and completion dates for each year group. There was no difficulty in gaining recruits because many students were looking for extra clinical practice experience. This is evident in the reasons given for their desire to participate, such as ‘I believe this will be for the betterment of nursing and an ideal way to improve personal nursing skills’, and ‘This is the most excited and motivated that I have felt since the beginning of the course. I am desperate to get into this program’ (Gonda et al. 1997).

Academic Preparation

The three academics involved in the first pilot were Kay, Karen and I, so no preparation was really required. However, we divided up our responsibilities. I was responsible for the support and evaluation of 1st and 2nd year students, Karen was responsible for the 3rd year students and Kay assisted and took control of negotiations and liaison among all of us.

Membership Characteristics/Roles and Responsibilities

As Edgecombe described in Chap. 2 (this volume), there were many participants in the development and implementation of the DEU, starting on the unit itself, extending to hospital administration, and then to the University academics and administrative staff. Each group is described below.

Participants Within the DEU

Nurses

There were many RNs and ENs who had been employed in the unit for in excess of 5 years, some of whom had been nursing for more than 20 years. These nurses were also very experienced at educating students in the clinical environment and on the whole, even at this early stage of the DEU, they were committed to making it work.

Principal Academics (PA)

The three academics involved in the first pilot were also very experienced nurses and academics. All had been part of the nursing profession for more than 20 years. In addition, they had all been involved in the tertiary education of nursing students for more than 8 years and were passionate about clinical education. Their work in the DEUs was above and beyond the work expected of them in their roles as lecturers, but because they were aware that clinical education was at a crisis point, they were willing to devote the extra time.

The Clinical Nurse Consultant (CNC)

Like many of the nurses on the unit and the academics, the CNC was highly experienced in nursing and had been actively involved in clinical education of a variety of health science students for many years. He consistently encouraged education to be one of the top priorities on ward 5G, and this culture of education trickled down to other nursing staff in the unit. He was aware that there were many faults with the status quo in clinical education at that time. Therefore, he was keen to find the best model of clinical education and to make ward 5G the best environment for nursing students' learning. He saw the DEU as an opportunity to achieve that goal.

Students

The students in the first DEUs were not your typical undergraduate nursing students. They self-selected to be in the DEU even though it required them to participate in clinical practice for a greater number of hours than other students in the course at that time, and they had to manage it around their usual class times. Overall, they were the high achieving, highly dedicated students who had distinction averages.

Participants Outside the DEU

Participants from outside the DEU were connected either to Flinders Medical Centre or the School of Nursing at Flinders University.

The hospital participants were the 5th Floor Associate Director of Nursing and the Ward Manager for 5G. Their focus was to ensure that appropriate processes were adhered to in relation to the placement and supervision of students, from the hospital management perspective. Once the decision to go ahead with the pilot was made, they had little to do with its day-to-day implementation.

The University participants were the topic coordinators for the three clinical practice units: Kay, Karen and I.

Lines of Communication

In the first pilot, we did not overtly consider formal lines of communication. Most communication occurred informally but more formal lines developed over time. Informal lines of communication, for example, were those between the CNC and academics who communicated regularly whenever the academics visited the ward.

More formal communication occurred in meetings every 2 weeks between nurses on the ward and the academics. These meetings took place in the double staff time so as many nurses could attend as possible. During these meetings, any problems that had arisen as a result of the DEU were discussed. Student progress was also a major item of discussion.

In addition, the usual formal written communication occurred between the University, the hospital and the ward in relation to the allocation of specific students for clinical placements.

Resources

At this point in time, few resources were dedicated to the DEU beyond those provided for any clinical placements utilised by the School of Nursing at Flinders University.

The academics participating in the project offered their time above and beyond their usual workloads, as did the Clinical Nurse Consultant. The academics also donated some of their textbooks to the ward for student use.

DEU Steering Committee

At the end of Semester 1 of 1997, there was a general consensus among the implementation team that the DEU was progressing relatively well and had definite potential. Therefore, it was decided in collaboration with the Directors of Nursing (DON) from the Southern Health Care Providers to expand the pilot project to include wards from other health care agencies in the Southern district of Adelaide, South Australia. As a result, a formal Steering Committee was set up. In addition to the implementation team, this committee comprised a representative from each of the following health care agencies in the Southern area: Repatriation General Hospital (RGH), Noarlunga Health Service (NHS), Flinders Medical Centre (FMC), Royal District Nursing Service (RDNS) and Adelaide University (UA).

This group met on a regular basis to provide advice to the team and to oversee the implementation of the continuation of the pilot project.

The Flinders University Dedicated Education Unit Pilot Implementation Phase 2

Phase 2 of the pilot project was implemented in Semester 2 of 1997. In this phase, the Steering Committee decided to increase the number of DEUs to four and to spread them over three health care agencies. Another ward at FMC (ward 6D), a ward at the RGH (ward 1) and a combination of a medical and surgical ward at NHS were all recruited. Kay and Karen moved to be the PAs for two of these wards,

Kay for 6D and Karen for ward 1. Another academic from Flinders University, Ailsa n'ha Winifreyda, became the PA at NHS. This meant that I remained the sole PA on ward 5G at FMC.

Preparation of clinicians and academics and recruitment and preparation of students occurred in the same way as in Phase 1. The characteristics of these three groups of participants were also the same.

In addition, all aspects of the structure and processes of DEU implementation that had been used in the Semester 1 pilot were maintained. The only difference was the student numbers. Feedback from the 5G pilot indicated that there were too many students in the unit, so it was decided to reduce the numbers from 36 to 32. However, numbers on ward 1, 6D and NHS were determined based on the numbers of beds, patient acuity and the RN-to-patient ratio in each unit.

Inclusion of a Liaison Nurse

Feedback about the Semester 1 pilot from the ward staff of 5G and the CNC Peter Mason indicated that there needed to be a person in place to manage the students in the ward and to liaise with the PA about the students. Therefore, it was decided to create a new position—the liaison nurse (LN). The role of the person in this position would be to:

- Act as liaison:
  - For students between ward staff and the PA
  - With CNC re the ward needs
  - With ward staff re students' role, function and progress within the DEU
  - With PA re student progress
- Organise student experiences in routine nursing care:
  - Allocate students to RNs, student peers and patients
  - Arrange student rosters and liaise with the PA
- Anticipate and organise extra experiences for students in relation to their patient's care and in collaboration with the RN supervising the student, i.e. endoscopy clinic, stoma therapy, theatre and community agencies.
- Provide orientation days:
  - For 2nd and 3rd year students on their first day (i.e. a maximum of 4 days per semester)
  - Meet with 1st year students each morning to establish learning objectives
- Organise the accreditation of students in certain skills, as required by the health care agency and in collaboration with the PA, i.e. blood glucose testing.
- Maintain a record of student attendance.
- Assist the CNC and PA with written evaluations of student progress as necessary.

- Encourage other staff members to participate in student teaching.
- Take direct responsibility for the supervision of one or two students each shift.

(Proposal for RN to CN Upgrades in DEUs 1999: 2–3)

The LN position was viewed and promoted as a staff development opportunity for experienced RNs working in the unit. It was also decided that the person who filled this position would be determined by a collaboration of the PAs from the University, the DEU CNC and nursing administration from FMC, RGH and NHS.

The LN positions were advertised requesting applicants to submit an expression of interest to their CNC. Interviews were staged on each DEU with the DEU PA and CNC acting as interviewers.

Successful applicants were chosen for each of the DEUs and promoted to CN (level 2 RNs) for the period in which students were placed in the ward for the following semester. The School of Nursing remunerated each health care agency for the cost of this position upgrade.

Inclusion of University-Based Workshops

In Phase 1 of the project, clinicians were informed about the DEU concept at unit-based meetings. In Phase 2, it was decided it would be beneficial for clinicians from each of the units to attend these sessions simultaneously and that offering workshops on the University campus would best achieve this. Therefore, several introductory workshops were offered on a variety of dates to allow as many nurses as possible from each DEU to attend. These nurses were paid their usual salary to attend the workshop and the health care agency was remunerated so they could backfill to staff the units. Workshops covered topics such as:

- The concept of a DEU
- An overview of the Flinders University Bachelor of Nursing Course
- Assessment requirements and tools for each year level
- Peer teaching/learning theory and strategies
- Use of the *ANMC Competencies* (ANMC n.d.)

Feedback at the end of Phase 2 indicated that nurses who had attended these introductory workshops requested advanced workshops for those who were experienced with DEUs. Therefore, in subsequent semesters, advanced workshops were also offered under the same financial conditions. A little later, LN workshops were also offered, covering topics such as:

- How to deal with difficult students
- Clinical teaching strategies
- Providing constructive critical feedback
- Developing clinical learning contracts

Numbers attending these workshops increased every semester as the DEUs increased. Feedback was always constructive and positive. The workshops enhanced the sense of partnership between all members of the DEU collaboration. Participants were provided with Certificates of Attendance for their professional portfolios, which added to the sense of partnership and reciprocal valuing of clinical and academic staff.

Pilot Evaluation and Outcomes

Evaluation of the pilot project occurred continuously over the two semesters. In Semester 1, an independent research assistant conducted and transcribed focus group interviews with student and nurse participants from the DEU. The findings from these interviews informed the development of a qualitative survey questionnaire that was implemented in Semester 2.

A report was prepared for the Flinders University School of Nursing and the DEU Steering Committee at the end of the pilot project. It indicated that there were many advantages of the DEU and two disadvantages, as illustrated in Table 4.1.

Recommendations from the report were that the pilot should be extended for a further semester and a feasibility study be implemented with a view to introducing the model for the whole School. Other strategies suggested were:

- A restructure of the curriculum around the DEUs
- Provision of administrative support
- An evaluation of the outcomes of these strategies

Table 4.1 Advantages and disadvantages of the Flinders University pilot DEUs

Advantages	Disadvantages
Students had more time to practise and develop their skills	Students complained of too heavy a workload
Students learned from each other and whilst teaching others	
Students had a sense of belonging in the ward	
Students developed professional relationships with clinicians	Academics complained of too heavy a workload
Nurses had one group of students for an entire semester, overcoming the problems associated with having several groups for short periods	
Nurses were also able to develop their roles as clinician educators	
Academics felt less marginalised in the ward area	
Academic skills and knowledge were utilised to their best advantage in the context of real practice	
Research possibilities were available to both academics and nurses, and the opportunity for collaboration was evident	

Post-pilot Development

In Semester 2 of 1998, the number of DEUs was increased again, this time to seven, with six of these in acute care medical/surgical wards. However, in this semester a very different DEU was included—the Accident and Emergency (A & E) department at FMC. The idea was to test whether the DEU model could be adapted for a variety of different health care environments.

At the same time, I conducted a feasibility study to determine the 'appropriateness for all undergraduate nursing students at FUSA, School of Nursing preparing for registration' (notes of Clinical Teaching Mull held on Friday, May 25, 1998).

The conclusion of the feasibility study was that:

> ... moving to a predominant DEU model for undergraduate clinical placement in the Bachelor of Nursing at FUSA is feasible from an educational, service and staffing perspective. However, modification of the curriculum will be required to address the issue of workloads for students and academics .... (Gonda 1998: 5)

At about the same time, Karen Wotton and I were successful in gaining a small internal Flinders University grant to evaluate the outcomes of the DEUs. The research was designed using the themes developed from the previous evaluations implemented in the preceding year (Gonda et al. 1999) to generate a quantitative survey tool to ascertain the perceptions of clinicians, academics and students participating in the DEUs. This instrument consisted of a brief demographic section and 18 statements representing broad conceptual areas of the impact of the DEU on the ward, student knowledge and skills, staff teaching and learning, the PA role and students' relationships (Wotton and Gonda 2004).

A total of 300 questionnaires was mailed to clinicians, students and academics who were participants in the seven DEUs (including the A & E DEU at FMC), resulting in a response rate of 77 %. Student respondents ($n = 121$) consisted of all 3 year groups and clinician respondents ($n = 127$) included RNs and ENs. Academic responses ($n = 7$) were not included due to their small sample size (Wotton and Gonda 2004).

The results confirmed those of the previous evaluations. They showed that DEUs were perceived to have a number of positive effects in relation to student skill development and relationships between students and nurses and between nurses and academics. Of particular importance was that this clinical education model allowed academics, students and clinicians to ground theory introduced in the University in real practice and provided an opportunity to evaluate the relevance of such theory to practice (Wotton and Gonda 2004).

This study's outcomes and the *Feasibility Report* conclusions convinced the School that the DEU model had positive outcomes. The School Board, led by Professor Judith Clare, who had supported the pilot project throughout, made a formal decision to implement the DEU as the primary model of clinical placement for undergraduate nursing students.

Curriculum Development

In order to attend to the recommendation of the feasibility report that curriculum change was required to address the workload issues associated with the DEUs, many changes were made to its structure and processes over several months. These included:

- Semesters being stretched from 13 to 16 weeks to reduce the student weekly workload. This was achieved by using the extended semesters previously developed for the Flinders University School of Medicine as a benchmark in the proposal to Faculty and University Boards, by which it was subsequently approved. Stretching the semester allowed us to structure the course so that the same amount of content was delivered but with less face-to-face contact for students and academics on a weekly basis.
- All elective subjects being offered as intensives at the beginning of semester instead of throughout the semester. This resulted in students having to attend lectures, tutorials, etc. for less subjects in the weeks when they were attending the DEU.
- The timetable being structured for two distinct cohorts in each year group. One cohort was timetabled to attend University on Mondays and Tuesdays and to undertake their DEU practice on Thursdays and Fridays. The other cohort did the opposite. All students attended their University lectures on Wednesdays.
- Clinical learning objectives for all subjects were written so that they were overtly transferable to all clinical settings, including community, acute, mental health and operating theatres. This strategy allowed students to attend specialty areas of practice in whatever subject they were undertaking at that time.
- When the succeeding curriculum was developed shortly after the implementation of the DEUs, it was also driven by, and founded on, professional practice-based learning objectives.

In addition to all these strategies, a new academic position was created within the School, the *Manager: Dedicated Education Units*. This position was created to monitor and maintain the existing DEUs and to develop and implement new DEUs so that all students in the Bachelor of Nursing could be placed in DEUs. I was fortunate to be the first person appointed to this position by the Dean of Nursing, Professor Judith Clare. I remained in the position for the next 5 years, when, with great sadness, I left Flinders University.

Changes to the Flinders University School of Nursing Culture

As could be expected, the introduction of the DEUs created much cultural change within the School. This change was very stressful for some people, but for others, it was a time of excitement and an opportunity for transformation. Open, transparent communication was essential. This took the form of regular informal conversations and formal seminars and workshops with School faculty covering all aspects of DEU implementation. The workshops in particular were utilised as a venue for receiving feedback, clarifying issues and allaying fears. Over the 5 years that I managed the DEUs, the School culture changed in many ways, such as:

- It went from having approximately eight academics in 1997 regularly attending clinical units to facilitate students on their practicum to 22 (including sessional lectures) in 2003. In fact, most of the lecturers in the School participated.
- The academics who were PAs in DEUs included senior lecturers, associate professors and professors, whereas previously this was usually expected only of associate lecturers and lecturers.
- Recruitment of all academics into the School of Nursing included an expectation of clinical expertise required for the School at that time.
- There was an expectation of clinical facilitation of all new faculty.
- The development of a clinical professorship.
- Teaching became increasingly grounded in practice.

The consequence of this was a change in the relationship with the health services industry, as evidenced by:

- Increased research opportunities for both academics and clinicians
- Opportunities for joint conference presentations and publications
- Increased collaboration re curriculum and student assessment
- Development of mutual valuing and respect

From 1998, the DEUs developed exponentially from the original 7 to 35 over a 5-year period. In addition to acute hospital-based units, DEUs included:

- Community drug and alcohol services
- Private community dialysis units
- Royal district nursing services
- Emergency departments
- Operating theatre suites
- Palliative care
- Aged care
- Rehabilitation nursing services

Confirmation of the DEU's attributes came from outside the School in 2002 when a number of reports cited the DEUs as exemplars of best practice in clinical education for undergraduate nurses. Reports included the *National Review of Nursing Education–Our Duty of Care* (Heath 2002), the *Commonwealth of Australia Senate Inquiry into Nursing* (Australian Parliament et al. 2002) and the Australian University Teaching Committee (AUTC) *Final Report* (Clare et al. 2002). A Joanna Briggs Institute systematic review of clinical placement models identified the

DEU as a model that facilitated higher levels of student satisfaction as well as collaboration between universities and clinical facilities (Lockwood 2003: 31). This review highlighted that student satisfaction was consistently considered a valued outcome of clinical education.

Conclusion

By the end of 2003 when I left Flinders University to move to Brisbane, approximately 650 Flinders University undergraduate nursing students were placed within DEUs. Initially, it was hard work to recruit new units, but word of mouth and publication of two papers about the DEUs in 1999 (Edgecombe et al. 1999; Gonda et al. 1999) turned this around. Clinical units started to approach the School to initiate the set-up of DEUs in their organisations, and influential people from other universities visited Flinders University to observe the DEUs in action. Laurie Grealish from Canberra University was one of the first of these, as was the Head of the School of Nursing from Portland University at that time, Terry Miller. The outcome of these visits can be found in other chapters in this book.

References

ANMC. (n.d.). *ANMC competencies*. Australian Nursing and Midwifery Council. http://www.nursingmidwiferyboard.gov.au/Codes-Guidelines-Statements/Codes-Guidelines.aspx. Accessed 16 Aug 2012.

Australian Parliament, Senate Community Affairs References Committee, Crowley, R. C., & West, S. (2002). *The patient profession: Time for action. Report on the inquiry into nursing* (Parliamentary Paper 306). Canberra: Australian Parliament.

Clare, J., White, J., et al. (2002). *Curriculum, clinical education, recruitment, transition & retention in nursing*. Final report (pp. i–xiv, 1–376). Adelaide: Flinders University School of Nursing and Midwifery.

Edgecombe, K., Wotton, K., Gonda, J., & Mason, P. (1999). Dedicated Education Units 1: A new concept for clinical teaching and learning. *Contemporary Nurse, 8*(4), 166–171.

Gonda, J. (1998). *Report on feasibility of moving to a predominant DEU model for clinical placement in the undergraduate nursing programme*. Adelaide: Flinders University School of Nursing.

Gonda, J., Wotton, K., & Edgecombe, K. (1997). *Dedicated Education Unit pilot study report: The implementation and evaluation of a collaborative clinical experience model*. Adelaide: Flinders University School of Nursing.

Gonda, J., Wotton, K., Edgecombe, K., & Mason, P. (1999). Dedicated Education Units 2: An evaluation. *Contemporary Nurse, 8*(4), 172–176.

Heath, P. (2002). *National review of nursing education 2002: Our duty of care* (pp. 1–293). Canberra: Australian Government.

Lockwood, C. (2003). *The effectiveness of undergraduate clinical placement, models, methods and meaningfulness for key stakeholders in South Australia* (pp. 1–38). Adelaide: Centre for Evidence based Nursing South Australia, The Joanna Briggs Institute.

Mattessich, P. W., & Monsey, B. R. (1998). *Collaboration: What makes it work. A review of the literature on factors influencing successful collaboration*. St. Paul: Amherst H. Wilder Foundation.

Proposal for RN to CN Upgrades in DEUs. (1999). *Internal documentation* (pp. 2–3). Adelaide: Flinders University School of Nursing.

Wotton, K., & Gonda, J. (2004). Clinician and student evaluation of a collaborative clinical teaching model. *Nurse Education in Practice, 4*(2), 120–127.

Chapter 5
The Canberra Dedicated Education Unit

Kasia Bail, Donna Hodgson, Alan Merrit, Jo Gibson, Jan Taylor, and Laurie Grealish

Education is not the filling of a pail, but the lighting of a fire

—William Butler Yeats

Glossary of Terms in Order of Appearance in This Chapter

Dedicated Liaison Nurse (DLN) an experienced Registered Nurse (RN) selected from the practice area who takes on extra responsibilities, including overseeing clinical learning in the DEU and liaising between staff, students and academics/faculty; the liaison between the unit and the University (equivalent of the Liaison Nurse [LN] in the original Flinders University DEU)

Principal Academic (PA) an academic lecturer in clinical (nursing school faculty member) who visits the clinical setting prior to student placement to

K. Bail (✉)
Faculty of Health, University of Canberra, Canberra, ACT, Australia
e-mail: Kasia.Bail@canberra.edu.au

D. Hodgson
Mental Health Nursing Programs coordinator, ACT Government, Canberra, ACT, Australia
e-mail: Donna.Hodgson@act.gov.au

A. Merrit
Former Teacher at University of Canberra, Canberra, Australia
e-mail: amerritt@anmac.org.au

J. Gibson
Canberra, ACT, Australia
e-mail: JGibson@anmac.org.au

J. Taylor • L. Grealish
Faculty of Health, University of Canberra, Canberra, ACT, Australia
e-mail: Jan.Taylor@canberra.edu.au; laurie.grealish@canberra.edu.au

K. Edgecombe and M. Bowden (eds.), *Clinical Learning and Teaching Innovations in Nursing*, Innovation and Change in Professional Education 10,
DOI 10.1007/978-94-007-7232-8_5, © Springer Science+Business Media Dordrecht 2014

facilitate clinical staff preparation for working with the students and thereafter visits the clinical setting regularly throughout each semester; communicates and liaises with students, the LN and the CNC, and utilises their ongoing expertise to facilitate students' learning

Inservices staff and student professional development/capacity building strategies undertaken in the clinical environment

ANMC Competencies Australian Nursing and Midwifery Council competencies required for registration as a nurse (RN) or midwife (RM) (ANMC n.d.)

Assistant in Nursing (AIN) certificated nurses (not RNs) providing support to the nursing teams in clinical settings under supervision of RNs

Introduction

Canberra is the capital city of Australia, sitting within the Australian Capital Territory (ACT). Canberran health services support a population of 500,000 from the ACT local region, and the University of Canberra (UC) offered the only nursing degree based in Canberra up until 2006. UC has an undergraduate nursing student population of approximately 500 nursing students requiring over 15,000 clinical days.

As part of requirements with the regulatory body in the ACT, UC reviewed the undergraduate nursing curriculum in preparation for the 2003 accreditation. The 2003 review brought about changes to the curriculum, which was the starting point for a change in clinical design. The review identified that clinical education needed to further address collegiality between students, clinical staff and academics; student accountability for delivered care; and academic presence in the clinical areas. The Dedicated Education Unit (DEU) model utilised at Flinders University was identified as suitable and was implemented in 2003 following a one-semester trial in the acute sector (Grealish and Kaye 2004; Owen and Grealish 2006). The DEU was then expanded gradually and collaboratively to community, aged care and mental health settings.

Curriculum Design

The undergraduate nursing curriculum at UC is 3 years, with six semesters of prescribed nursing programme, with each semester containing a clinical subject. The nursing curriculum is clinically focused, with emphasis on the development of critical thinking and reflection. Class work and assessment are designed to scaffold students using clinical practice to understand theory, and theory to understand

Table 5.1 UC nursing students' clinical learning experiences

Year/Sem	Days per week, commencing	Total days in field
Year 1, Sem 1	1 day a week from Week 10–14	4 (plus 10 clinical workshops prior to field placement)
Year 1, Sem 2	2 days a week from Week 10–14	8
Year 2, Sem 1	2 days a week from Week 5–14	16 (no clinical during W8 and 9)
Year 2, Sem 2	2 days a week from Week 5–14	16 (no clinical during W8 and 9)
Year 3, Sem 1	2 days a week from Week 2–14	24 (no clinical during W8 and 9)
Year 3, Sem 2	3 days a week from Week 2–14	34 (no clinical during W8 and 9)

practice. Learning is seen as a social experience, and the development of nursing identity is an important underpinning of undergraduate education. Consequently, there is an emphasis on the feedback students gain in both clinical and theoretical components of their learning, and how it 'feeds forward' to affect their professional development.

Part of the curriculum redesign was in reshaping the timing of clinical placements to privilege clinical equally with the theory of classroom work. This meant moving away from isolating clinical in block placements into an integrated model in which students go on placement in each semester of the programme, starting in Semester 1 of first year and increasing the amount of time spent in placements as they progress through the course. This facilitates structural integration of theory and practice on a weekly basis, as shown in Table 5.1.

The purpose of implementing DEUs was to:

- Increase students' clinical exposure
- Offer students greater continuity and stability in their clinical learning environment
- Enable students to be in the unit for the full shift, be held accountable for care provided and be considered part of the nursing team
- Promote learning in clinical environments
- Facilitate the integration of theory and practice
- Acknowledge the role of the clinician in student learning and provide greater opportunities for clinician involvement
- Strengthen clinical/University links and collegial relationships
- Promote positive experiences for staff and students
- Provide the opportunity for student peer learning, support and modelling in the clinical environment

Who's Who in the Canberra Dedicated Education Unit

The DEU is a collaborative set-up, and the model is designed to maximise the strengths of the nursing unit within which it sits. Consequently, there may be clinical staff or manager leadership roles in addition to those described here. Also, some of the nomenclature for similar roles within the University of Canberra and Flinders

University DEUs is slightly different. For example, the University of Canberra uses the term Dedicated Liaison Nurse (DLN), whereas Flinders University uses the term Liaison Nurse (LN).

All DEUs have at least one Dedicated Liaison Nurse (DLN), nominally a level 1 RN from the clinical area, upgraded to a level 2 by the University. The DLN maintains a clinical load and is also responsible for liaison with clinicians, students, senior nurses and academics regarding the DEU. A Principal Academic (PA) spends 4–10 h a week within the DEU, with additional time taken for planning, liaison and meeting with students on campus. The PA is primarily responsible for clinical assessment of the students and is a teaching member of the University, usually convening other units in the undergraduate curriculum. The DLN and PA roles in the UC DEU are similar to the LN and PA roles in the original Flinders University DEU, as described by Gonda (Chap. 4, this volume).

In the DEU, assumptions are made that each student is individual; is interested in becoming a nurse; wants to perform well; is responsible for their own learning; requires guidance in how to question practice, where to find information and how to practise; and has a complex personal life.

Students can learn from observation of, and engagement with, the clinicians in tasks, team work, patient, family and multidisciplinary communication—students talking about practice and nursing work are learning.

Expectations of clinicians as learning facilitators in the DEU are that clinicians: are employed to care for patients/clients; have valuable expertise that can be shared in a range of ways; learn from engagement in nursing work; have valuable observation and assessment skills; can provide students feedback and 'feedforward' (suggestions about what else the student might need to think about, read about or practice are important); and have a professional responsibility to support student learning.

Clinicians work closely with students on each shift as part of their normal caseload. They may be allocated a number of students and may need to organise work using a team nursing model to accommodate those students. Clinicians support student learning by allocating them work within their scope of practice and receiving reports/feedback on patient activity from students throughout the shift. Clinicians are expected to share concerns about students' progress with the students and appropriate staff as soon as possible.

How the Dedicated Education Unit Supports Learning

The DEU model provides an opportunity for students to become immersed in nursing practice. Learning in the DEU is not only about attaining clinical skills; it is also concerned with how nurses work with their patients/clients, with the broader health care team and with each other. Thus, learning occurs equally within the patient interactions and the tea room. The social elements of the DEU are very powerful in allowing the students to develop a nursing identity.

At a structural level, the Canberran DEUs are similar in that they work to create a community of practice, sharing knowledge and learning from each other. Common features include:

- Student numbers are approximately 24 per DEU, although the size of the DEU in terms of beds, nurses or location varies.
- DEUs are managed collaboratively through 'Reference Groups', with representations from academics, clinicians and students, who meet between one and six times a year.
- Each DEU is evaluated each semester by the Reference Group and through surveys.
- Other health professionals as well as nurses make important contributions to student learning and are considered part of the community.
- Some DEUs or areas within DEUs are 'rested' once every few years depending on staffing needs.

Function of Canberran Dedicated Education Units: Learning Activities

Students at each DEU are supported to identify their own learning goals for the clinical placement. Many students struggle with this initially, often focusing on the skills that will be available on that particular placement, for example, blood glucose levels (BLG) on an endocrine ward or wound dressings in the community. Students realise personal areas for development as they become immersed in practice experiences and set goals related to these experiences. Students are encouraged to make the most of any incidental activities that occur while they are on the clinical unit, for example, inservices, multidisciplinary case conferences, patient transfers or procedures or allied health interventions. These incidental activities, which help students to make links between the health system and patient trajectories, are more easily accessible because students are in the areas for a significant period of time and seen as part of the team.

PAs and DLNs may facilitate feedback from clinicians to students. Sometimes feedback forms are used to prompt clinicians to give more detailed feedback. Shadowing or coaching, where the PA or DLN facilitates discussion between staff and students on the ward, can help provide more encouragement for the activity.

PAs and DLNs can use different activities to promote learning. Often, students are asked to present a patient case to their peers in a group debrief facilitated by the PA, thus demonstrating knowledge about pathophysiology, medication, nursing care and communication. Students may also research particular topics of interest and present these to peers in formal settings or informally as part of the teams' work. Students are supported to access the health facilities' policies and procedures and any other health informatics relevant to the workplace. Sometimes students' academic workload includes a presentation of their in-class assignments as an inservice to the ward staff. The assignments are designed to integrate students' clinical experience with theory and thus are directly relevant to the clinicians with whom the students are working. For example, a student designed a flip chart to inform patients/clients about machines in operating theatres ('Machines that go Bing'). Another student researched handovers and presented information about the different purposes and requirements of the nursing handover.

Assessment

Students are supported to self-assess as a component of their formative assessment part of the way through their placement. Students are provided with the Australian Nursing and Midwifery Council (ANMC) *Competencies* (utilised for registration of nurses in Australia) and asked to describe examples where they have demonstrated components of nursing practice, such as 'practices within an ethical nursing framework' or 'establishes and maintains therapeutic relationships'. The students self-assess performance against the standards, utilising the Bondy Rating Scale (1983). Formative assessment is provided informally in meetings with the PA and/or DLN and includes discussion, feedback and feedforward. The PA and/or the DLN conduct summative feedback, which is part of the final assessment. This is again graded against the *ANMC Competencies* (ANMC n.d.) using the Bondy Rating Scale. The final assessment takes place at a meeting with the student and is based on three major sources of evidence: student self-assessment, PA judgement on attitudes and knowledge based on critical conversations over the semester and specific feedback about clinical skills and attitudes from clinicians with whom the students have worked. This ongoing summative assessment contributes to progressive learning across placements throughout the students' degree. The meeting also has a formative aspect, and students are encouraged to identify their learning needs for the next months of their careers.

How Clinicians Are Engaged in the Learning Culture

The DEU is a service unit dedicated to learning, but whose learning is not specified. The model acknowledges that once individuals are involved in questioning behaviour, the local group, not just the individual who asked the first question, engages in opportunities for discussion and practice development. In addition to the above structures and learning activities, clinicians may also be supported through:

- Regular contact and conversations with an academic about current clinical ideas
- Opportunities to engage in research (e.g. Boogaerts 2004; Boogaerts et al. 2004, 2008; Grealish and Kaye 2004)

- Informal and formal education from the PA, including:
  - Student education on specific topics as needed
  - Clinician education through discussion about current practice and research
  - Discussion about ethical issues
  - Current practice or national developments
  - Discussion about standards or scope of practice (students and staff)
  - Inservices given by the PA, either related to teaching/learning (e.g. giving and receiving feedback, peer learning, the DEU model, adult learning, the UC curriculum) or to the PA research specialty (e.g. prognosis communication)
- Feedback forms, designed to develop clinician and student feedback participation skills
- Evaluation survey, to gain feedback from clinicians about the performance of the DEU, PA and DLN
- Orientation involvement, where the clinical area designs how they would like to introduce students to their area
- 'Mega DEU', where once a year all DLNs and DEU clinical managers are invited to a forum as an opportunity to develop collaboratively and learn from each other
- Twice-yearly free workshops for clinicians working with health students on clinical placements, provided by UC
- Involvement of students and academics at ward team meetings
- Debriefs and liaison with staff regarding student support/behaviours
- Local developments as invited, for example, staff recruitment or practice development working party

Acute, Multisite and Distributive Models of DEUs: Benefits and Challenges

Eleven DEUs were functioning in the ACT by 2009. These were across community, public, private and mental health settings and took the form of three different models. They were not designed differently initially but evolved differently during collaborative ventures between UC and the different health facilities.

Acute Setting

The six acute settings of the Canberran DEUs include medical and surgical wards (in both public and private hospitals), paediatrics and operating theatres. In an acute DEU placement, students will often move across locations within the hospital, following their patients/clients' journeys.

Multisite Setting

There are two DEUs in Canberra functioning across multiple sites. The multisite setting is identified by primary leadership of a PA, with supportive contacts in each site that has either organisational or specialisation ties. One setting is the Residential Aged Care Facility (RACF) DEU, which comprises four individual facilities, one PA and leadership from the nurse educators or Directors of Nursing at each facility. (For more information on the Residential Aged Care Facility DEU, see Grealish et al. 2010.) The second setting is an Aged Care and Rehabilitation Service (ARCS) DEU, which includes a rehabilitation ward, acute aged care ward, residential aged care units and a rehabilitation step down unit, one PA and four facility educators functioning as DLNs.

Distributive Model: Mental Health and Community Care

The leadership and championing of the DEU ideals are distributed amongst individuals and across locations in the Distributive DEU model. Canberra utilises two unique DEU settings that facilitate learning in the community and mental health sectors, which operationalise the Distributive model. While community and mental health are growing and essential components of the health system, clinical placements for nursing students remain predominantly hospital-focused. Finding ways to integrate these aspects of nursing into the curriculum is important for nursing education, as well as recruitment, and for improved client and community outcomes. The Distributive model is effective in generating a culture of learning across an organisation. Much of the PA work includes interagency liaison and student support in order to establish a network of student-friendly workplaces. Student group debriefs allow presentation of focused information relevant to current issues and for students to share experiences across the different areas. Students gain additional awareness of the patient trajectory as they access a wide range of providers in these Distributive models.

The Community Care DEU has 24 sites and four programmes, three directors, eight nurse managers, five CNCs and approximately 300 RNs and ENs. The DEU is facilitated by one PA who works closely with a group consisting of one DLN and representatives from each of the programmes.

The Mental Health DEU has in excess of 12 clinical sites with three different health care providers and approximately 25 DLNs. The PA works closely with the DLNs and other clinicians and students as the need arises.

Reflections

Research exploring perceptions of the DEU model in the ACT has found that students accept the responsibility for their work and learning in the DEU and value that responsibility. Students value peer learning for sharing experiences, reinforcing knowledge and enhancing confidence (Ranse and Grealish 2007). Clinicians report that working with students is a worthy investment of time and effort, where students' fresh eyes, recent knowledge and questioning behaviours contribute to their workplace. Clinicians also see students as a future investment; educating and supporting them now provides nurses for the future (Grealish et al. 2010).

The 'Dedicated' nomenclature in the DEU title initially described a unit committed to the nursing students of only one University. However, most of the DEUs in Canberra have students from other education providers. Over time, the 'Dedicated' part of the title has grown to describe a clinical unit that is 'dedicated to learning', rather than dedicated to only one particular group of students. The 'Dedicated' nomenclature also reflects the clinical areas' commitment to students' learning. Many areas have developed their own initiatives to foster their own roles for education in the unit, often foregoing the level 1 to level 2 payment incentive for a DLN. The 'Dedicated' nomenclature can also be attributed to the academic who is dedicated to that DEU.

Student and clinician feedback has articulated some of the strengths of the DEU models in the different settings. Nurses report that having so many students at once (up to five on any one shift) just makes them part of the nursing work, so monitoring their progress and needs is on your 'nursing radar' in the same way as the patients/clients. Nurses also find that students help with the nursing work and the nurses miss them when they've gone. This is not just about tasks but about critical inquiry and making suggestions to improve ward function. Some nurses attribute this to the 'fresh eyes' students bring to their workplace and the process of their inquiry.

A strong component for student enthusiasm for the model is that they feel part of the team, responsible and relied upon. Students are able to take on a gradual patient load, from sharing care for one patient to being the primary carer for four or more patients/clients. Students value the opportunity to make human connections and build communication skills, including amongst their peers. Students work closely with a range of clinicians, finding role models across disciplines. Also, they gain both organisational and patient trajectory knowledge as they engage in the local events for the teams within which they are working. Recruitment opportunities occur due to this engagement, either as Assistants in Nursing (AIN) while studying or when returning as graduates.

Challenges for the DEU include some that affect other models of clinical placement. Workplace stressors of changing skill mix and staff turnover at times impact upon clinician and student needs. A DLN with a good working knowledge of clinicians' strengths, and who can evaluate student needs throughout the semester and match people together as best as possible, is very valuable.

At times, students feel they are 'working, not learning'. Hughes (1998) has described 'the perils of the authentic workplace'. In the DEU, work with the DLN and PA is needed to explore the relationship between work and learning and in identifying student goals and how students can reach them. The DLN, PA and clinicians, by facilitating clinician-to-student feedback, set the context for students to maximise learning opportunities. Clinicians need support to provide constructive criticism to students, even when students specifically ask how they can improve. A challenging component of the clinician and student relationship is working with borderline/unsatisfactory students. Helping clinicians distinguish between students 'doing the work' and knowing the 'what and why' requires development of suitable learning structures to enable critical questioning of students by PAs, DLNs and clinicians.

Finding out how to adapt the DEU to different health facilities requires ongoing revision and engagement. For example, Reference Group attendance was low in one setting. An adapted model of leadership was required with one-to-one meetings between the PA and clinical leaders to maintain consensus and operation. Another example was managing the sheer number of students in small, clinical spaces in the acute setting. Encouraging students to be aware of space issues and to prioritise the patients/clients' and nurses' needs was effective in reducing the extent of the issue. Another example was supporting students in aged care to understand roles in working with AIN and Enrolled Nurses (EN). Students needed guidance in identifying how they could work with AIN and EN and understanding the workforce structure and culture.

A particular administrative challenge with the DEU is organising police record checks, immunisation, uniforms, identification cards and orientation for 1st year students or students transferring into the course because students go on placement so early in their first year.

Conclusion

The Canberran DEUs have been running for 7 years, with a range of clinical locations and models of practice. The DEU, as a model of clinical education, provides a contemporary framework for clinical learning, facilitated by clinicians at their clinical venue and supported by academic staff on site. The Bachelor of Nursing course has undergone and continues to undergo significant revision. There is now a greater focus on clinical learning, where students engage in learning about nursing work by doing nursing work; the physical and emotional experience, as well as cognitive understanding, leads to learning. In this model, learning is the student's responsibility and is facilitated by clinicians. The academic presence in the clinical learning environment brings information about the curriculum, supports students and clinicians in questioning taken-for-granted assumptions and, where possible, engages the clinicians in practice development. Student, academic and clinician feedback has been predominantly supportive of the DEU and indicates that this model promotes learning of both students and clinicians, facilitates integration of theory and practice and enables collegial linkages between the University and clinical facilities.

References

ANMC (n.d.). *ANMC competencies*. Australian Nursing and Midwifery Council. http://www.nursingmidwiferyboard.gov.au/Codes-Guidelines-Statements/Codes-Guidelines.aspx. Accessed 16 Aug 2012.

Bondy, K. (1983). Criterion-referenced definitions for rating scales in clinical evaluation. *Journal of Nursing Education, 22*(9), 376–382.

Boogaerts, M. (2004, November 3). *Student experiences in Community Health Dedicated Education Unit*. Oral presentation, ACT Health, Community Health Nurses Symposium: Learning—Doing—Connecting, Canberra.

Boogaerts, M., Dane, M., & Grealish, L. (2004, November 25). *Back to the future: Introducing undergraduate nursing students to the community setting*. Oral presentation, Australian Council of Community Nursing Services Colloquium, Brisbane.

Boogaerts, M., Grealish, L., & Ranse, K. (2008). Policy and practice: Exploring tensions to develop practice. *Practice Development in Health Care, 7*(1), 49–57.

Grealish, L., & Kaye, L. (2004). Change and challenge: The implementation of a new model of clinical learning for undergraduate nursing students in a cancer setting. *Australian Journal of Cancer Nursing, 5*(2), 3–4, 6–7, 9–11.

Grealish, L., Bail, K., & Ranse, K. (2010). Investing in the future: Residential aged care staff experience of working with nurses in a 'community of practice'. *Journal of Clinical Nursing, 19*(15–16), 2291–2299. doi:10.1111/j.1365-2702.2009.03133.x.

Hughes, C. (1998). Practicum learning: Perils of the authentic workplace. *Higher Education Research & Development, 17*(2), 207–227.

Owen, J., & Grealish, L. (2006). Clinical education delivery. A collaborative, shared governance model provides a framework for planning, implementation and evaluation. *Collegian, 13*(2), 15–21.

Ranse, K., & Grealish, L. (2007). Nursing students' perceptions of learning in the clinical setting of a Dedicated Education Unit. *Journal of Advanced Nursing, 58*(2), 171–179.

Chapter 6
An American Experience: Transition to the Dedicated Education Unit Clinical Education Model

Carol Craig and Susan Randles Moscato

Glossary of Terms in Order of Appearance in This Chapter

University of Portland UP

Clinical Faculty Coordinator (CFC) nursing faculty from the University who plans students' experience and informs Clinical Instructors (CIs) what is covered in University classes each week

Magnet facilities/hospitals hospitals awarded recognition by the American Nurses Credentialing Center (ANCC) as demonstrating excellence in nursing care

Clinical Instructor (CI) a staff nurse who wants to teach

Lead Teacher academic staff in charge of both lecture and clinical components of a clinical course; responsible for assigning grades

Chief Nursing Officer CNO

School of Nursing SON

Oregon State Board of Nursing OSBN

Nurse Manager selects the staff nurses to become CIs, works closely with the CFCs about CI, student, and system issues on the unit, and arranges CI staffing assignments so they are present on student clinical days

Clinical Educators CE

National Council Licensure Examination (North America) NCLEX

C. Craig (✉) • S.R. Moscato
School of Nursing, University of Portland, Portland, Oregon
e-mail: craig@up.edu; srmoscato@gmail.com

K. Edgecombe and M. Bowden (eds.), *Clinical Learning and Teaching Innovations in Nursing*, Innovation and Change in Professional Education 10,
DOI 10.1007/978-94-007-7232-8_6, © Springer Science+Business Media Dordrecht 2014

Introduction

In the USA, developing, growing, and evaluating academic-practice partnership processes and outcomes are coming of age. DEUs have taken this lead, demonstrating how successful partnering not only optimizes clinical nursing education but also optimizes collaboration and improves quality care on patient care units with the goal of enhancing student outcomes. Prior to 2003, clinical teaching at the University of Portland (UP) was done in the traditional American model: one faculty with 8–10 students to teach, monitor, support, and evaluate. On an acute care hospital unit, the faculty or charge nurse assigned patients to students, and the staff nurse who was caring for the patient would have the student follow behind them. The staff nurse, at their discretion, delegated tasks or had the student observe. Usually the staff nurse would not know the student's abilities, learning needs, knowledge base, or expectations. The instructor often would have students placed on different units and would divide time among the units and students. Students would wait for their instructor to be with them to perform different skills. A typical clinical day would be filled with waiting and observation rather than performing care. Instructors had little chance to observe the student's communication and critical thinking skills. Staff nurses might have little interest or skill in teaching, and students dreaded hearing staff comments such as "I have a student *again?*", "Oh, no, we have students today," or "The students are wearing purple. It must be Tuesday."

Faculty at UP were aware of the limitations of the current model, but also of two key issues in the larger environment: the shortage of nurses to provide care and the shortage of nursing faculty. Schools of nursing in Oregon were challenged to increase the number of graduates despite a dearth of faculty. When faculty and administration became aware of the Dedicated Education Unit (DEU) model in Australia as an innovation in nursing education, they decided to explore the model and its potential for effective clinical education in our program. As illustrated in this chapter, the UP DEU made several adaptations to the Flinders University DEU model to meet the particular needs of the curriculum and clinical placement contexts. One notable difference is the use of block-style placements in the UP model. The UP DEU also uses a very different nomenclature from that used in both the Flinders University (Chaps. 2 and 4, this volume) and Canberra University (Chap. 5, this volume) DEUs, reflecting how different academic and clinical nursing environments require roles designed to suit them.

Implementing the First University of Portland Dedicated Education Unit

Establishing a DEU was a slow and deliberate process. The keys to a successful DEU lay in relationships, identification of mutual goals, and open, ongoing communication. Agency administration at the highest level must support the process, and clinical staff and faculty who will be working together to educate the students must get to know one another through collaboration to establish trust. In addition, the state Board of Nursing must agree to regulatory support, even if only on a pilot basis.

The first step at UP was to approach the top nursing administrative leader at a clinical partner facility in a health care system that had a long history of affiliation with the University. The nurse executive agreed with the concept and gave it her full backing. She selected the first units to pilot the DEU. This support provided an entry for the University to continue the discussions with Nurse Managers and then with staff nurses. Only when the Nurse Managers were on board and had chosen the staff nurses who were early adopters to lead the transformation was it possible to move forward, a process that took many months of meetings and many hours of discussion. A parallel process was ongoing at the University, in which faculty discussed their role in a DEU and agreed to try the new model. The Board of Nursing was involved from the beginning of the process and actually encouraged both the agency and the University to be innovative.

Basic assumptions that underlie the innovation were developed mutually to guide the first DEUs. The assumptions were modified as the agency and UP worked together and the DEU concept matured through lived experience. The current DEU assumptions are:

1. The DEU provides an optimal environment for faculty and clinical nursing staff to cultivate mutual respect, develop partnerships, and appreciate the skills each brings in educating students in the best possible way.
2. The primary purpose for the DEU is to improve the quality of clinical education in an efficient and effective manner as a response to the nursing shortage. It is expected that a school using the DEU concept will require fewer units for clinical instruction because of the model's efficiency.
3. Only students from one school of nursing will be on a DEU at a time. The School of Nursing faculty member will be called a Clinical Faculty Coordinator (CFC) and will serve as a coach for the staff nurses on the unit. The CFC will not be expected to be on the unit at all times students are there but will be available electronically at all times.
4. When the students on a DEU are Bachelor of Science in Nursing (BSN) students, Clinical Instructors on the unit will be prepared at the BSN level whenever possible. The expert nursing skills of all nurses who are interested in teaching are recognized and valued on the DEU.
5. It is an expectation that all professional nurses, especially those in Magnet facilities, will contribute to the education of the next generation of nurses.
6. Nurses on the DEU will be prepared and supported in their teaching role by the academic partner.
7. A DEU in concept does not need to be one unit; it could be multiple units.
8. Students may be placed around the clock and 7 days a week to maximize the ability of staff nurses to become Clinical Instructors. Patient assignment for Clinical Instructors on the unit varies with the students' skill level.

9. Patient satisfaction and clinical quality are expected to remain stable or improve.
10. Clinical Instructor, student, and faculty satisfaction will be better than under previous teaching methods. Clinical Instructors look forward to students and experience joy in the teaching role rather than seeing teaching as a burden.
11. The preceptor role is elevated to that of Clinical Instructor, recognizing the professional development and passion for teaching of those who most wish to teach.
12. It is the Clinical Instructor's (CI) responsibility to engage in critical conversations with students to help assure continued growth while meeting the educational outcomes expected in the clinical setting.

These assumptions underscore the concepts of partnership, the unit as an optimal learning environment and quality nursing outcomes. The assumptions also make it clear that the entire unit, not just individuals on the unit, creates a village so that it "takes a village to educate a student."

Roles and Responsibilities

Once agreement was reached that the unit would become a DEU, the work of deciding each person's crucial roles and responsibilities began. The major roles within the DEU were agency administrators, University administrators, Nurse Managers, Clinical Faculty Coordinators, Clinical Instructors, and a Lead Teacher. The responsibilities they undertook are outlined in Table 6.1.

Timeframe

Establishing the DEU took time. It took about a year from the idea to opening the unit as a DEU. Even now, with the model well-articulated and the roles and responsibilities established, the preferred timeline is about a year to establish a new DEU. As can be seen in Table 6.2, many decisions need to be made, and some structural changes may be necessary.

Stakeholder meetings held at the beginning of the process should include everyone who might be concerned with the DEU; even those who might be considered "peripheral" to the unit, such as nurses with float positions and managers of other units who may be asked to provide support, housekeepers, physical therapists, and ward clerks. Establishing the unit as an educational place means not only getting dedicated space for students but also getting materials for the unit staff. Finally, even after the DEU has been launched, "Celebrations of Partnership" are needed to continue the close relationships upon which the DEU depends. Quarterly

Table 6.1 Major roles and attendant responsibilities in UP DEUs

Role	Responsibilities
Agency administrators	Supplied strategic vision but also agreed to be flexible with budget and staffing needs for the new unit
University administrators—School of Nursing administrative team	Provided oversight for the model, budgets for coordination meetings and Clinical Instructor (CI) orientation and training
	Chose faculty for Clinical Faculty Coordinator (CFC) positions
	Worked with the Board of Nursing to write a demonstration project for board approval
Nurse Manager	Selected the staff nurses who became CIs and worked closely with the Clinical Faculty Coordinators (CFCs) about CI, student, and system issues on the unit
	Arranged for CI staffing assignments that would allow them to be present on student clinical days for 6-week blocks of time (a typical rotation)
Clinical Faculty Coordinator (CFC)—the pivotal role in the UP DEU model. Considered the "lynchpin" for the success of the DEU, the CFC is the essential bridge between the agency and University at the unit level. The CFC is a UP faculty member who usually holds a Master's degree in nursing and is considered an expert teacher by the University administration	Acted as the liaison between the University and the CIs
	In each unit, the CFC mentored the CI in best teaching practices, helped the CI to support and challenge student learning, provided continuing education to the CI for teaching/learning, posted the student classroom topics and learning needs each week, and worked with the Nurse Manager to solve problems
	The CFC did not work directly with the students when they were on the unit providing care, but ran weekly student seminars that brought the learning into the bigger picture
	The CFC, with the CI, evaluated student learning. The CFC reviewed student paperwork, collaborated with CIs to address student learning needs, and assigned the clinical grade
	The CFC met with the CI at least once during a clinical day to discuss CI teaching needs or student learning needs. The CFC was not present on the unit all the time the students were working but was available 24/7 by cell phone should a critical incident occur

(continued)

Table 6.1 (continued)

Role	Responsibilities
Clinical Instructor (CI)—the nurse who provides the expert, at-the-bedside teaching for students under the supervision of the CFC. This nurse usually has a baccalaureate degree in nursing, but occasionally a CI will have an associate or diploma degree in nursing. Both levels of nurses have at least 2 years of experience and are considered clinical experts by their Nurse Managers before they are selected to be educated for the CI role	Provided the clinical teaching to the student
CIs are encouraged to allow students to do appropriate care themselves, rather than to observe the CI provide care	Each CI had two students for 2 days per week over a 6-week period. The shifts varied in length from 8 to 12 h. Therefore, a CI knew the student well and was able to allow the student to participate fully in patient care, supporting the student when needed
	The CI helped the students to integrate theory, practice, and research and challenged the students' clinical reasoning
	Provided extensive feedback to the CFC about student progress and learning needs and worked with the CFC to guide and develop student learning
	Sought out clinical experiences for the student to integrate and support classroom learning
Lead Teacher—the faculty in charge of both lecture and clinical components of a clinical course	Responsible for class design
	Provided the classroom discussion and oversight for course outcomes—provided the syllabus to the CFC and reviewed evaluations of the CIs and CFCs on the unit
	Assigned the course grade for the overall course, which at UP is a combination of classroom and clinical grades

meetings, which are organized and funded by UP, are dinner social meetings and include unit management, CFCs, and University administrators. "Lunch & Learn" in-service presentations are organized each semester for the CIs to help develop teaching/learning skills. The network of relationships remains as important as the day-to-day work between CIs, CFCs, and students.

Table 6.2 Sample Dedicated Education Unit timeline for implementation

	Spring	Summer	Fall	Spring
Beginning of stakeholder meetings				
Dean and CNO commit to exploring partnering to open a DEU	X			
SON consults with Board of Nursing (regulatory agency) about use of the DEU model	X			
Unit and unit manager selected as potential site of the DEU—support from agency education department secured	X			
Unit manager and SON deans meet to explore the DEU concept for the unit and initiate "buy-in" by staff	X			
Unit meeting with staff organized by unit manager to further explore idea—SON representatives attend	X	X		
Follow-up on meeting with Nurse Manager and SON representatives—identification and buy-in of "early adopters"—discuss research potential and begin the internal IRB discussions	X	X		
Socializing begins—staff meetings, emails, flyers, community building with SON associate deans/directors, CFC, and staff	X	X	X	
Unit-based activities to prepare for conversion to DEU model				
Decision to become a DEU—date set for launch (e.g., first rotation of the semester)		X		
Structural changes to accommodate students—DEU classroom designated and reserved, locker room space (backpack bin) for students designated, computer access arranged and extra computers acquired, reference books donated by SON, SON paraphernalia distributed and displayed		X	X	
Clinical Instructors (CIs) attend all-day CI orientation on campus—topics of orientation include SON philosophy, program outcomes, clinical reasoning model, DEU roles and responsibilities; teaching/learning strategies; and practice/debrief in the simulation lab. CIs complete paperwork for OSBN and receive DEU CI handbook			X	
CFC meets with Nurse Manager and "early adopter" CIs to continue planning for launch. First day clinical day orientation planned for students including computer training planned. Mechanism for ongoing problem solving and communication selected		X	X	X

(continued)

Table 6.2 (continued)

	Spring	Summer	Fall	Spring
Launch of DEU—3 CIs each with 2 students—arrangements made for reduced patient assignment for the CIs at launch			X	
Debriefing sessions held with CIs and Nurse Manager			X	X
Ongoing communications with CIs, Nurse Managers, and CFCs to problem solve and manage change to the new clinical teaching model		X	X	X
Mid-rotation student evaluations—CI and CFC coordination with student			X	X
End of rotation student evaluations–CI and CFC coordination with student; students write "thank you" letters and evaluate the CIs, CFCs summarize student evaluations and write CI evaluation, send to CI and copy to NM for file; CIs complete an on-line evaluation of the CFC			X	X
New 6-week rotation begins with another set of CIs and students			X	X
Supports for DEU success				
Monthly meetings with CFCs and Associate Dean	X	X	X	X
Quarterly meeting of CFC, NM, facility nurse educators, deans on campus for dinner	X	X	X	X
"Lunch & Learn" teaching/learning CE sessions presented each semester by CFC for CIs	X	X	X	X
Celebrations of Partnership—Ongoing appreciation activities from the University [adjunct faculty theater passes, masseuse on unit, food and flowers]			X	X

SON School of Nursing, *OSBN* Oregon State Board of Nursing, *CI* Staff nurse DEU orientated Clinical Instructors, *NM* Nurse Managers, *CFC* Clinical Faculty Coordinators (University Faculty), *DD* Deans and Directors from University, *CNO* Chief Nursing Officer

Challenges

The biggest challenge was to maintain clear and consistent communication between the agency and UP because we work in different worlds with different schedules and different priorities. Some faculty were concerned about the idea of losing the traditional Clinical Instructor role. They worried about maintaining high quality in-clinical instruction and whether they would become redundant in the School of Nursing. Faculty knew that their paperwork would increase with a larger number of clinical students, and that they would be challenged to push the students to a higher level of understanding rather than the completion of tasks. Faculty found it uncomfortable to be mentoring staff nurses about teaching rather than supervising student practice. Faculty also had to develop a trust in the CIs to evaluate students appropriately.

Staff nurses were concerned about workload, and whether they could do patient care and closely supervise two students at the same time. The increased number of students who would potentially be on the unit worried some staff nurses, who were also hesitant about whether they could be good teachers, and what they would do when they needed to manage a difficult student. Agency administrators were concerned about increased costs to the agency if staff nurses were given a reduced patient load for the first week or two of clinical instruction. These concerns were similar to those identified during the implementation of DEUs at Flinders University and Canberra University in Australia, as described in by Gonda (Chap. 4, this volume) and Bail et al. (Chap. 5, this volume).

Outcomes/Evaluation of the Dedicated Education Unit Model

The DEU model has worked very well with our students, faculty, and agency partners (Moscato et al. 2007). The agencies have benefited from efficient use of existing resources and the nurses' professional development. The University has benefited from quality clinical education of increased numbers of students. Both have benefited from the recognition of the model as an excellent recruiting and retention tool. Individuals working at the agencies and University reported other advantages in using the model, as described in the following text.

Clinical Faculty Coordinator Feedback

Clinical Faculty Coordinators (CFCs) found the DEU role rewarding and reported that the change gave them an innovative model for practice. The CFCs had a new ability to provide higher level interactions with students, with a greater focus on critical thinking than on skills or tasks. The clinical paperwork load needed to be closely monitored so that CFCs were not overwhelmed with grading and evaluation. Their relationships with staff nurses gave them a greater appreciation and understanding of the challenges and opportunities nurses face in day-to-day practice, along with a realization that the CIs provide very high quality clinical instruction and feedback to students.

Staff Nurse Feedback

Staff nurses found it was very possible to supervise two students while providing care and enjoyed being a team. The synergy of collective learning enhanced care. As the unit evolved into a learning community, the increased numbers of students were not problematic. CIs grew in confidence as they experienced their new role as teachers and reported excellent support from the CFCs in working with difficult students and challenging learning situations.

Student Feedback

Student feedback on the DEU has been positive. Students appreciate working with a single nurse who knows their capabilities and learning needs. The close contact with a staff nurse allowed them to be more efficient and effective. They felt like part of the unit rather than an intruder. Students reported taking the lead on patient care rather than merely observing care. They also did not spend time waiting for an instructor to be with them for new skills or high-risk procedures. Most students preferred the experience of the DEU to the traditional model.

Magnet Hospital Status

A "Magnet" hospital is one that has been awarded recognition by the American Nurses Credentialing Center as a hospital that demonstrates excellence in nursing care (ANCC 2010a). The original 14 "Forces of Magnetism" include nursing leadership, participation in education and research, and quality of care and nursing autonomy (ANCC 2010b). The 14 forces were incorporated into a model in 2008 that shows the dynamic relationship between them (ANCC 2010b).

An important Force of Magnetism is the requirement that nurses are teachers. The DEU has been cited as an example of teaching excellence in the decision to grant Magnet status. Part of the teaching excellence is that students who are not meeting clinical expectations are recognized earlier and intervention activities can be initiated earlier. If a student is not able to meet the clinical objectives, the DEU model provides consistent clinical observations and records to help students achieve desired outcomes or to make the case for course failure or dismissal from the program. All three of the hospitals that have UP DEUs have now achieved Magnet status, and the DEU model was commended each time as an exemplar of excellence.

Faculty and Nurse Shortage Outcomes

Changing from a traditional model to a DEU meant that all senior students and about half the junior students could be educated within a DEU for their medical-surgical experience. Student numbers increased threefold over this time, so that each year UP graduates went from 80 per year to just over 220. The number of agency units required went from 25 to 7. Clinical faculty numbers did not increase for the medical-surgical clinical experiences. UP faculty estimated that the University would need 20–25 paid faculty and 26–80 practice units to manage this number of students in a traditional model. The faculty to student ratio would be 1:8 or 1:6 but would involve more units because most units would only accommodate 2–4 students. The model has also been essentially budget neutral for the agencies, as slightly increased costs during clinical were offset by slightly decreased costs during orientation following hire.

Students also maintained high pass rates on the National Council Licensure Examination (NCLEX). First-time pass rates are benchmarked at 92 % and, except for an aberration in 2007, have all been at 92 % or higher since inception of the DEU.

Increased Professionalism

A number of the nurses chosen to be CIs were inspired to grow into new roles. The "rigor of sharing goals with professional colleagues" (Warner and Burton 2009: 333) resulted in some remarkable professional outcomes as practice informed education and education influenced practice. CIs stated that teaching enforced their clinical skills and gave them a role model as educators. They stated that they found satisfaction in their relationships with students and the ability to influence the next generation. They found that their contact with CFCs helped them to see new models for scholarship and practice. There is committed agreement by CIs that "we will never go back to the old way." CIs certified as expert clinicians gave scholarly presentations and assumed leadership roles on the unit. Some returned to school for a Master's degree or have been promoted into a leadership position within their hospitals. For example, one of our CIs is now a Nurse Manager of the unit. She credits her teaching role as a CI for the impetus to go back for her Master's degree, which in turn led to her promotion to a manager position. UP and agency administration called this "positive turnover," since the nurses stay within the agency but in higher positions.

Latest Innovations

The DEU model can be done in many different care settings (Moscato et al. 2013). To date, UP has 7 DEUs on medical-surgical units, 1 DEU on a psychiatric unit, and 3 DEUs in long-term care facilities (LTC). The LTC DEUs use a new clinical model in which students will be assigned to a team consisting of a certified nurse assistant, an RN, a charge nurse, a social worker, and a physical therapist. The students work with the team to provide care and learn the many facets of long-term care. The goal is to provide practice in basic nursing skills as well as the ability to admit, provide discharge planning, understand rehabilitation therapies, and work with physicians to provide care for patients in rehabilitation and long-term care.

Conclusion

Relationships remain the key to the successful implementation of the DEU model. Establishing a DEU requires building close working relationships with agency administration, management, and frontline staff. Maintenance of a DEU requires ongoing communication between agency partners and the University on many levels. The process takes time and can be laborious, but the rewards are numerous in terms of faculty, staff, and student satisfaction with clinical education.

References

American Nurses Credentialing Center. (2010a). *Forces of magnetism*. http://www.nursecredentialing.org/Magnet/ProgramOverview/ForcesofMagnetism.aspx. Accessed 4 Apr 2011.

American Nurses Credentialing Center. (2010b). *Announcing a new model for ANCC's Magnet Recognition Program*. http://www.nursecredentialing.org/Magnet/ProgramOverview/New-Magnet-Model.aspx. Accessed 12 Nov 2011.

Moscato, S., Miller, J., Logsdon, K., Weinberg, S., & Chorpenning, L. (2007). Dedicated Education Unit: An innovative clinical partner education model. *Nursing Outlook, 55*, 31–37.

Moscato, S., Nishioka, V., & Coe, M. (2013). Dedicated Education Unit: Implementing an innovation in replication sites. *Journal of Nursing Education, 52*, 259–267 (available online April 2013).

Warner, J. R., & Burton, D. A. (2009). The policy and politics of emerging academic-service partnerships. *Journal of Professional Nursing, 25*(6), 329–334.

Chapter 7
Dedicated Education Units: Christchurch Polytechnic Institute of Technology and Canterbury District Health Board (CPIT/CDHB), New Zealand

Michelle Casey and Deborah Sims

Glossary of Terms in Order of Appearance in This Chapter

Christchurch Polytechnic Institute of Technology, New Zealand CPIT

Registered Nurse (RN) college or University qualified nurse licensed by a nursing registration body to undertake all facets of nursing in accordance with the body's regulations

Canterbury District Health Board, New Zealand CDHB

Clinical Liaison Nurse (CLN) an experienced RN selected from the practice area who takes on extra responsibilities, including overseeing clinical learning in the DEU and liaising between staff, students and academics/faculty (particularly the ALN); the liaison between the unit and the University. Role comparable to the LN in the original Flinders University DEU model and the DLN in the University of Canberra DEU model

Edited by Jane Mountier [CPIT research assistant]; reviewed by Members of the DEU Working Group (Dr Cathy Andrew RN, BA, MA(Hons), Ph.D., MCNANZ, Head of Nursing School, CPIT; Mary Gordon, CDHB Executive Director of Nursing; Rose Whittle RGON, AdvDipN(CP), BA (Ed.), Plunket Cert, Applied Science Cert, School of Nursing Clinical Leader/ Principal Lecturer; Raelene Shaw CDHB DEU governance group; Deb Cook RN, Cert Clin Tchg, MN Lecturer, Clinical Co-ordinator; Isabel Jamieson RN, BN, MNurs(Melb), CertAT, Senior Lecturer. All from CPIT and CDHB, New Zealand).

M. Casey (✉)
Canterbury District Health Board (CDHB), Christchurch, New Zealand
e-mail: Michelle.Casey@cdhb.health.nz

D. Sims
Christchurch Polytechnic Institute of Technology (CPIT), Christchurch, New Zealand
e-mail: Deborah.Sims@cpit.ac.nz; simsd@cpit.ac.nz

K. Edgecombe and M. Bowden (eds.), *Clinical Learning and Teaching Innovations in Nursing*, Innovation and Change in Professional Education 10,
DOI 10.1007/978-94-007-7232-8_7, © Springer Science+Business Media Dordrecht 2014

Academic Liaison Nurse (ALN) a permanent clinical lecturer at the University who provides consistent support to students and clinicians

Charge Nurse Manager (CNM) similar to the Nurse Manager role in the Portland DEU, takes responsibility for 'appointing' a RN to the Clinical Liaison role (CLN) and rostering time for preparation, orientation and assessment as well as attendance at staff development/capacity building sessions

Introduction

Prior to 2006, the model of clinical teaching and learning for undergraduate Bachelor of Nursing (BN) students at the Christchurch Polytechnic Institute of Technology (CPIT) centred on the preceptorship model of individualised one-on-one support, provided by experienced Registered Nurses (RNs) from within the clinical environment. Preceptorship has long been regarded as the 'gold standard' model of supporting undergraduate nursing students in clinical learning environments (Budgen and Gamroth 2008). In this model, academic staff (clinical lecturers) visit intermittently to provide curriculum integration and to monitor the student's progress with the student and their preceptor. The academic staff could be full time, part time or casual. Anecdotal evidence and emerging data from within the CPIT School of Nursing and the Canterbury District Health Board (CDHB) identified factors thought to be impacting on the successful implementation of one-on-one preceptorship, including:

- The inability of undergraduate nursing students to 'mirror' the rostered-rotating shifts undertaken by RNs.
- Preceptor absence from the clinical environment due to sickness, study or annual leave.
- Fluctuating demands of the clinical environment.
- Increasing number of RNs working part time.
- The impact of casual 'hospital pool' or outside agency staff on each area.
- CDHB staff's limited knowledge and understanding of the BN programme.
- Perceived 'invisibility' of the CPIT clinical lecturer.
- Issues around student assessment. In some cases, students were working with different preceptors on a regular basis, resulting in a lack of consistency in experiences and expectations and difficulty collating data for student assessment purposes.

These factors were the impetus for establishing Dedicated Education Units (DEUs) for CPIT undergraduate nursing students.

Changing the Status Quo: Establishing the Dedicated Education Unit as the Preferred Model of Clinical Teaching and Learning, 2006–2008

A report on undergraduate nursing education in New Zealand noted that 'DEUs are a good example of a model in which students work shifts alongside registered nurses but do so in a collaborative and supportive environment in which clinicians and educators work together' (KPMG 2001: 88). Following a visit to Flinders University in Adelaide to consult with key stakeholders about the concept and benefits of the DEU model of clinical education, CPIT and CDHB signed a Memorandum of Understanding for establishing a pilot DEU model.

The Canterbury Dedicated Education Unit Pilot Model Project

The initial project was undertaken by a Project Team whose brief was to investigate the possibility of establishing a DEU for CPIT nursing students undertaking clinical placements within the CDHB and identify the advantages and disadvantages of this model compared to the existing preceptorship model. The Head of School, Nursing (CPIT) and Executive Director of Nursing (CDHB) sponsored the project. However, a 'bottom-up' approach was utilised with 'top-down' support. Both organisations supported DEU Project Team members' time to commit to the project. A Governance Group was created to oversee the introduction of the DEU (see example Fig. 11.2 in Edgecombe et al. (Chap. 11, this volume)).

The research project aimed to:

- Document the process of trialling DEU pilot sites through action research
- Evaluate the model's suitability for the local context and its ability to support undergraduate nursing students undertaking clinical placements
- Make recommendations to the Governance Group about the suitability of the DEU model for use as an ongoing clinical education model for CPIT students undertaking clinical education in CDHB placements

The CPIT Ethics Committee approved the project in June 2007. Over the next 12 months, the DEU Project Team and Governance Group worked to shape the Canterbury model and develop a research proposal. During this time, the Project Team undertook extensive marketing of the DEU model and pilot project. They developed DEU branding, brochures, communication strategies and workshop content and defined roles and responsibilities. Education sessions were presented to senior nurses at Canterbury's three tertiary teaching hospitals outlining the DEU pilot project, its aims and evaluation process; the DEU model; the key roles of Clinical Liaison Nurse (CLN), Academic Liaison Nurse (ALN), staff and students; and a proposal on how it may work in reality.

Practice areas were invited to submit an expression of interest if they wished to be part of the pilot project. Initial plans were for three DEU pilots but five areas indicated their willingness to commit to the process.

Action Research

Action research was recommended because it would enable systematic exploration of the situation (Street 2004) and afford opportunities for cycles of action that promote change. It was also most suited to the collaborative, practice-orientated and context-specific nature of the DEU pilot project because it would offer co-researchers (the Project Team) and participants (the ALNs, CLNs, DEU staff and students) a collaborative approach to making improvements to, and fostering their understanding of, their practice environments (Cardno 2003). In addition, it would support and enhance relationships between participants and co-researchers.

It was not possible to adhere strictly to a pure action research methodology due to the number of clinical areas involved and the number of staff working in the DEUs. However, the three-phase Cardno and Piggot-Irvine Model (1994), which informed the project, included the following key action research concepts:

- The research focused on practical knowledge and strategies in a specific context.
- A systematic cyclical research process was used, allowing for change and improvement.
- Strong links were retained between research, action and evaluation whilst allowing for a shifting focus as required (e.g. at some times the research is foremost, at others implementing action takes priority) (Street 2004).

Development of New Roles

Adopting the DEU model required the development of two new roles: the Clinical Liaison Nurse (CLN) and Academic Liaison Nurse (ALN). The CLN is an RN selected from the practice area who takes on extra responsibilities, which include acting as a liaison person between staff, students and the ALN, arranging students' rosters, organising student learning experiences and gathering information from staff in order to complete student assessments in collaboration with the ALN. The CLN is provided with supernumerary time to attend a DEU workshop, prepare for the students' arrival, develop and run student orientation programmes and undertake students' formative and summative assessments. In this phase, the Project Team worked with pilot practice area DEU Charge Nurse Managers (CNM) to identify a suitable CLN for each DEU. The CLN role in the CPIT/CDHB DEU model is comparable to the Liaison Nurse (LN) in the Flinders University DEU model (Edgecombe, Chap. 2, this volume and Gonda, Chap. 4, this volume) and the Dedicated Liaison Nurse (DLN) in the University of Canberra DEU model (Bail et al., Chap. 5, this volume).

The ALN (formerly the Clinical Lecturer) is a CPIT permanent tenured or permanent part-time staff member allocated time to work with students as per usual CPIT processes. The ALN provides consistent support to students, staff and the CLN and works with the CLN on students' assessments. The CPIT Head of School, Nursing, selected the ALNs for each DEU.

Members of each pilot DEU, in conjunction with the Project Team, decided on a minimum of six students per clinical placement. Students were informed about the project, provided with information about the DEU model and allocated to DEUs via the established CPIT process.

Data Collection and Analysis

Focus groups, the CPIT Clinical Evaluation Tool (CET), research diaries and ALN and CLN personal logs were used to collect data during clinical placements between August and November 2007. This multi-method data collection facilitated triangulation. All focus group participants were provided with an information sheet and consent form prior to their involvement. Completion and submission of the CET questionnaire implied consent. Research assistants who were privy to raw data signed a Confidentiality Form.

Thematic analysis was conducted on the qualitative data collected from the focus groups, research diaries and comments from the CET questionnaire, firstly on each data set separately, then triangulated across these findings. Work logs were analysed by comparing the hours logged to the allocated work hours. Descriptive statistical analysis of the CET data was undertaken using Statistical Package for Social Sciences 15 (SPSS) (IBM n.d.). Two Project Team members not involved with the initial qualitative data analysis examined the findings from each data set with respect to consistency (a match between findings) and contrast (contradictory findings) to further establish rigour.

Findings

There were no significant differences in the data between the two cycles and no significant changes were made between them. There was a high degree of consistency within and between findings. Key findings from both data collection cycles were summarised into two major themes: supporting clinical learning and relationship building.

Supporting clinical learning was expressed by nursing students who valued the 'one-on-one teaching at the bedside [from the ALN]' because the ALN 'could see what we are capable of'. Students described the CLN as 'the one constant' or 'our rock' they could go to when they had questions or needed support with clinical decision-making. Students emphasised they felt welcome and part of the DEU team and valued being overtly acknowledged by interdisciplinary team members (Levett-Jones and Lathlean 2008; Levett-Jones et al. 2009). They credited 'really good orientation' for this, developed with input from both academic education and practice (Hale and Jamieson 2009; Jamieson et al. 2008), because it gave them more confidence to 'go out and join the team'.

Relationship building was evident when both ALNs and CLNs worked collaboratively to support students and DEU staff throughout the clinical placement. Students realised quickly that the ALNs and CLNs were 'working together on the same page'. One ALN described the CLN role as 'invaluable as support for ALN, pivotal, with communication and setting goals and standards, encouraging peers to enhance student independence/initiative'. The CLNs appreciated having the ALN to turn to for support with student issues, stating 'ALNs can deal with student issues straight away', and 'ALNs working with issues together with CLN'. The ALN was more visible in the DEU model, and DEU staff knew when the ALN would be in the practice area. The 'ALN had a timetable so everyone knew when they were coming in … important and not just dropping in'.

The results of the pilot project demonstrated that the DEU model could be established successfully within the local context of the CPIT and CDHB partnership (Casey et al. 2008). A copy of the full summation report is available online at: http://www.cdhb.govt.nz/deu/default.htm.

The Canterbury Dedicated Education Unit Philosophy

The pilot programme resulted in the articulation of a shared philosophy. The collaborative partnership between the education provider and the service provider allows practice areas to offer a supportive clinical learning and teaching environment for students. The following principles underpin the partnership between CPIT School of Nursing and a DEU practice area.

Dedicated Education Unit Principles: CPIT/CDHB

Shared responsibility and commitment to creating a learning partnership between education and practice.

Cooperate in an open and cooperative manner, share information, with meaningful consultation, networking, collaboration and support as the basis for the partnership.

Acknowledgement that each partner has different structures of accountability and each partner has the right as a separate entity to express their views independently.

Acknowledgement that partnership relies on common vision and commitment from partners at every level to achieve the collective aims. In doing so, partners recognise that decisions made within one organisation indirectly affect the other and neither can accomplish the combined purpose alone.

Management processes exist to monitor quality and report regularly to all partners regarding the outcomes of the partnerships.

Partners will demonstrate their commitment to each other and their mutual vision by adequately resourcing the partnership.

Implementing the Dedicated Education Unit Model in Canterbury: 2009–2010

On completion of the pilot programme, agreement was reached to establish DEUs within the CDHB region, and the implementation phase began. The Project Team became the DEU Working Group, and all members belong to the Governance Group, ensuring the Working Group receives direction and support from senior staff from both organisations. Terms of Reference for both groups were reviewed (a copy of the CPIT/CDHB Terms of Reference is included as Figs. 11.7 and 11.8 in Edgecombe et al. (Chap. 11, this volume, which illustrates step-by-step how to set up a DEU using the CPIT/CDHB process as a template)).

In April 2009, the Executive Director of Nursing (CDHB) seconded a Nurse Educator (NE) to support the implementation of additional DEUs and to work closely with DEU staff. The NE DEU is an original member of the Working Group and works closely with the School of Nursing clinical management team at CPIT, representing the CDHB on CPIT committees such as the School of Nursing's Clinical Practice committee. Currently the role is allocated 0.5 FTE (full-time equivalent) and has been vital in supporting new and existing DEUs. The role has grown over time to fit the needs of both organisations.

The Working Group has a changing membership but aims to have equal representation from education and practice. This has built many bridges between the partners and created a level of collaboration that extends far beyond the DEU model.

The vision, support and commitment of Directors of Nursing (responsible for nursing staff within a hospital), Nursing Directors (responsible for nursing staff within services) and Charge Nurse Managers have been essential for the success of the DEU model (Crawford and Whittle 2008). Key to the implementation of the model has been their continuing support for undergraduate nursing students in the workplace despite increasing demands to provide support to nursing students, interprofessional students and new graduate nurses. DEUs have been established in Medical/Surgical, Mental Health, Emergency Department (ED) and Community Health clinical contexts.

Key Roles in the Canterbury Dedicated Education Unit

The key roles in the DEU are the Clinical Liaison Nurse (CLN), Academic Liaison Nurse (ALN), DEU staff, students and the Charge Nurse Manager (CNM). A brief account of each role is given here. Full descriptions of roles and responsibilities can be found on the CDHB Internet site http://www.cdhb.govt.nz/deu/default.htm.

Clinical Liaison Nurse (CLN)

The Charge Nurse Manager allocates the role of CLN, using a checklist developed by the Working Group (see example Fig. 11.9 in Edgecombe et al., Chap. 11, this volume). Initial plans were for one CLN (1.0 FTE allocated to the role) per DEU, but experience has shown that two RNs role-sharing can be more effective. This gives each CLN more flexibility in their roster and reduces the workload associated with student assessment. It also supports succession planning by providing mentoring for nurses moving into CLN roles.

The CLN is responsible for student orientation to the DEU, arranging student rosters, allocating students to DEU staff/peers/patients and formative and summative student assessments. The CLN acts as a liaison person between students, DEU staff, the ALN and the Nurse Manager. CLNs are encouraged to work alongside each student at times throughout the placement. Their direct observation of the student's progress towards meeting learning outcomes contributes to the assessment process.

Feedback reported from a Medical/Surgical DEU, ED DEU and a Community DEU illustrates how students, staff, CLNs and ALNs viewed and valued the CLN role.

> The CLN role is the link between staff, students and the ALN. Students value this role and find it 'absolutely vital' because the CLNs 'were friendly and knew our names', were 'in touch with what the students were doing', 'alerted you to learning opportunities', 'had great knowledge and skills' and were 'great role models for students'. Students liked that the CLNs were familiar with the CPIT assessment forms and were supportive of the students. Students really appreciated 'just knowing there was one person you could go to, knowing she was there for us' and that she was 'always available' and 'always checked in, asked what was happening'.
>
> DEU staff valued the CLN role because it took the 'pressure off (assessment) for staff' and students 'got a fairer assessment because of the CLN role'.

The CLNs also commented that there was 'less stress for the RNs to have someone else doing assessments'. The ALN commented on how it was 'so incredibly fair having the CLN bringing feedback from staff' (*Feedback from the Medical/Surgical DEU*).

'I gather feedback from staff on student progress. Having the DEU system meant that staff could feedback anonymously' (*CLN, Emergency Department [ED] DEU*).

Academic Liaison Nurse (ALN)

The ALN is a permanent full-time, proportional or part-time member of the School of Nursing. In the past, casual staff were often used to support students in the clinical practice areas, with some areas having a different clinical lecturer each semester. An ALN who is familiar with the area can work alongside students in the practice setting, teaching and facilitating learning within the context of practice. ALNs are able to actively link theory to practice and directly observe students' progress towards meeting learning outcomes. ALNs contribute to orientation programmes, facilitate learning and perform formative and summative assessments. Feedback from students, ALNs and CLNs about this role in a Medical/Surgical DEU demonstrates its value in the clinical learning environment.

The ALN role provides academic support for students, who often commented that the ALN 'helped to link theory to practice' and asked many questions of them which 'would really make you think'. The ALN 'was an essential and pivotal role, providing an essential link between theory and practice'. Students also said the ALN role 'assisted us with goal setting, gave direction and helped us to use correct terminology–it was good to have the ALN there as we still had to do academic work'.

A big part of the ALN role is relationship building with students, the CLN, the CNM and staff in the DEU area. 'One of the advantages to being an ALN is having a more collegial relationship with the CLN and staff'. Also, 'when staff are comfortable giving feedback to me about students I feel chuffed about this'.

The CLN and ALN work together closely to support students. As one CLN said, 'the ALN role marries academic with practical. The ALN knows exactly where students are at and is supportive of them' (*Feedback from the Medical/Surgical DEU*).

'The CLN felt well supported by the ALN who was accommodating, on the ward regularly and was in regular contact via email. The ALN worked well with students and would discuss issues with the CLNs. This enabled problems to be dealt with appropriately and in a timely manner' (*Feedback from the Medical/Surgical DEU*).

DEU Staff

DEU staff facilitate student learning by actively involving students in the assessment, planning, provision, evaluation, documentation and reporting of nursing care. Staff contribute to creating a climate of positive support and mentoring for students; a climate in which students' presence is valued and their contribution recognised. They play a role in student assessment by giving feedback to the ALN and/or CLN on student progress. Staff are expected to demonstrate a high standard of professional and evidence-based nursing practice, along with a commitment to their own ongoing professional development.

It is vital that DEU staff are supportive of students whilst they are on clinical placement. Members of the multidisciplinary team are often introduced to students on orientation day and make an effort to find learning opportunities for students. Student feedback indicates that students find DEU staff helpful and welcoming.

'It's been so good to have staff support me and want us to be there' (*Student feedback Medical/Surgical DEU*).

'I've never worked anywhere where even the doctors would take us aside and teach us' (*Student feedback, ED DEU*).

'We were accepted into the team right away' (*Student feedback, Mental Health DEU*).

'Health care assistants were really knowledgeable and helpful' (*Student feedback, Medical/Surgical DEU*).

First placement students reported they worked with a variety of DEU staff and in general found that staff made them feel comfortable, were willing to answer questions, share knowledge and encourage them. Students liked working with different staff as they 'get to pick up different styles'. This helped students develop their own style of nursing. One student commented that it was 'good to work with someone who I did not connect with as I still learnt from them ... and this made me reflect on how nurses work'. Students felt that nurses would come and find them when teaching opportunities were available and that it was 'really good, would go in-depth with teaching stuff ... remembered how it was to be a student' (*Student feedback, Medical DEU*). Staff often 'looked for learning opportunities' for students and also 'looked for students if something interesting was happening' (*Student feedback, Mental Health DEU*).

Students

Larger numbers of students can be accommodated in the DEU practice areas. Each DEU has a minimum of six students who are expected to take responsibility for their learning and self-monitor their progress towards required competencies. Students receive support, feedback and ongoing evaluation of progress from the CLN, ALN and DEU staff. Collegial relationships with other students are expected and encouraged, using opportunities for learning as they occur. Students are encouraged to 'peer teach'. This can be formal or informal, depending on course requirements. Peer teaching occurs in an opportunistic fashion through informal discussion, case study presentations, practising skills together and observing each other. Students are sometimes unsure what peer teaching means and whether it has occurred. A common observation by students is that they have tapped into one another's knowledge 'by accident'. Students have reported in their feedback that it is good to talk to peers rather than other nurses because they can hear what peers have been doing and then 'go and have a look to see/try new things'. Some students also mentioned they would ask the 'stupid questions' of each other first to make sure the question was valid before going to the nurse (*Feedback from the Medical/Surgical DEU*).

Key Features of the Canterbury Dedicated Education Unit Model

The following key features of the Canterbury DEU model are inbuilt to ensure the model works in accordance with the previously stated DEU principles and evaluation of the pilot DEUs. These key features enable DEUs to adapt and operate successfully in different practice settings:

- The practice area is dedicated to supporting undergraduate nursing students on clinical placement.
- Students placed in a DEU will be supported by two key roles: the Clinical Liaison Nurse (CLN) and Academic Liaison Nurse (ALN).
- The CLN is a regular staff member of the practice area who has an interest in promoting and facilitating clinical learning for undergraduate students.
- The ALN is a tenured staff member of Christchurch Institute of Technology (CPIT) dedicated to a DEU practice area.
- All staff working within the DEU practice area support teaching and learning opportunities for undergraduate nursing students, e.g. registered nurses, enrolled nurses, nurse assistants, pool nurses, Medical and Allied Health staff.
- DEU staff are flexible and responsive to student learning.
- Education and practice organisations support, value and recognise the contribution that staff make to student learning.
- Students start placement with a structured orientation.
- Allocation of patient load should be commensurate with student's skill and ability.
- Patient/client allocation for CLN is taken into account by the Nurse Manager.
- CLN is the consistent person from DEU practice area who undertakes student clinical assessment and is a support for students and staff.

- Quality of patient/client care is paramount.
- Peer teaching and learning is encouraged and valued.
- Commitment to evidence-based practice, undertaking collaborative research, research utilisation and quality improvement.
- Staff committed to ongoing professional development.
- Teaching and learning are valued.
- Relationships are open and feedback encouraged.
- Acknowledgement that 'repetition' is essential for skills acquisition.
- Learning occurs through direction and delegation.

These key features enable DEUs to adapt and operate successfully in different practice settings, for example, in Medical and Surgical (hospital) wards, Mental Health Services or the Community setting, as illustrated in Table 7.1.

Recruitment and Education of Dedicated Education Unit Staff

DEU principles are incorporated when recruiting staff in the DEU practice areas. The Working Group facilitates workshops each semester to educate new CLNs and ALNs, CNMs and key nursing staff. The workshop also updates existing DEU staff on any curriculum changes, provides opportunities to problem solve any issues and challenges established DEUs to look for quality assurance and research opportunities within their areas. Some of the more established DEUs involve students in quality activities such as auditing care plans. Clinical teaching and learning strategies are introduced at the workshop, and participants are encouraged to share their own strategies. Time is allocated for key staff to meet. In new DEUs, this time is used to plan for the next semester, whilst in existing DEUs it is used for review, evaluation and discussion of innovative ideas.

Clinical Practice Diary: A Communication Tool

Following the pilot, the Working Group introduced the Clinical Practice Diary as a tool to assist with communication between staff and between students and staff (see example Fig. 11.10 in Edgecombe et al., Chap. 11, this volume). In an environment where students work alongside many nurses, the diary provides continuity and indicates to nursing staff the level at which the student may be working.

The student is encouraged to discuss and record their goals for each shift with their assigned nurse, then review these later in the shift for feedback on what went well and to identify areas to work on in the following shift. For example, a student has a preoperative patient one shift and would like to have the same patient the following shift to follow through patient care, thus becoming familiar with the patient journey.

Table 7.1 Examples of Dedicated Education Units in different practice settings

deu Supporting Clinical Learning®	Medical & Surgical DEU	Mental Health Service DEU	Community DEU
Student numbers (minimum 6)	10	11	7
Year of students	Years 2 and 3	Year 2	Year 3
CLN Role (1 FTE)	2 CLNs allocated to share the role	2 CLNs allocated to share the role	3 CLNs allocated to share the role
ALN Role	1 ALN allocated		
Orientation process	One day orientation provided primarily by CLNs with ALN input	One day orientation provided primarily by CLNs with ALN input	NE arranges and hosts orientation to the organisation with ALN input. It is difficult for CLNs to be involved
Peer teaching	Occurs informally through discussion and presentations to each other	Occurs informally through discussion, case study presentation, students working with each other and weekly supervision sessions	Occurs informally though discussion and group reflection weekly
Teaching and learning opportunities	Students spend time in a surgical orthopaedic unit, orthopaedic rehabilitation unit, operating theatre, post anaesthetic care unit, acute admitting and outpatient department	Students are allocated to an inpatient or outpatient area of the service. Those who are allocated to an outpatient area spend a few days in an inpatient unit	Students spend time in areas of hospice, wound clinic, IV therapy, acute nursing service, continence, stoma, diabetes
Rosters	Year 2 students work Monday–Friday morning (0700–1500) and afternoon shifts (1430–2300). Year 3 students work Monday–Sunday all shifts	Students work Monday–Friday morning (0700–1500) and afternoon shifts (1430–2300)	Students work Monday–Friday, normal working hours

(continued)

Table 7.1 (continued)

	Medical & Surgical DEU	Mental Health Service DEU	Community DEU
	Students receive the roster before placement The CLN is rostered supernumerary time in advance for formative and summative assessments	Students receive the roster before placement The CLN is rostered supernumerary time in advance for formative and summative assessments	Students receive the roster before placement The CLN is rostered supernumerary time in advance for formative and summative assessments
Assessments	CLN/ALN complete assessment together		
Staff feedback to CLNs/ALNs	CLNs actively seek feedback on student progress and performance from staff		
Research/quality activities	Students participated in audits and provided feedback on theatre placement	Students involved in audits and provided feedback on an admitting research tool	Students and staff identified several quality and research projects they had participated in or observed

Assessment

In the Canterbury model, students' formative and summative assessments are undertaken by the CLN and ALN. This process was introduced to promote the role of the DEU staff as clinical teachers and to provide a consistent and valid assessment process because students work with multiple nurses.

Each formative assessment is allocated 1.5 h. The student completes their self-assessment and gives it to the CLN or ALN the day prior to assessment. For the first 30 min of the meeting, the ALN and CLN discuss the student's self-assessment and their own estimation of the student's progress. The student then joins the meeting to discuss their progress and to set goals for the remainder of the placement. This documentation is completed within the 1.5 h time frame. Summative assessments follow a similar format, but only 1 h is allocated.

Feedback about assessment in different DEUs supports the validity of the assessment processes that have been put in place. A brief summary of feedback from

CPIT/CDHB DEUs illustrates how these processes enhance the positive experiences for students and staff in DEUs.

> Students complete a self-assessment first and then the CLN, ALN and student would go through the assessment together. Students reported that the 'interactions between ALN, CLN and staff [were] obvious' and 'enhanced learning during the assessments' (*Feedback from the Medical/Surgical DEU*).
>
> Students considered the assessment process 'positive' and 'fair', and both ALN and CLN had input and 'gave reasonings for their assessments' (*Feedback from the Surgical DEU*).
>
> Students appreciated that the CLN and ALN worked together on the assessment as the 'ALN knows more of the forms, academic ... the CLN knows practical ways to improve' (*Feedback from the Community DEU*).
>
> The assessment process was easy because I only needed to link/consult with the CLNs rather than multiple preceptors. In addition, I felt it was easy for the CLNs and me to reach a consensus on student progress when completing the assessment forms (*ALN feedback, Mental Health DEU*).
>
> An ALN felt that she really knew how the students were functioning when it came to the assessment due to 'the collaborative nature of working together with the CLN. Bringing the clinical and academic viewpoints together was the best part' (ALN f*eedback, Medical/Surgical DEU*).
>
> It is wonderful that we don't have to do assessment. We just enjoy the students (*Staff, Community DEU*).
>
> Staff feel more relaxed about having students because they do not do assessments. The environment is more supportive for students as staff and students know who is doing the assessment (*CLN feedback, Community DEU*).

Challenges

Whilst the DEU Working Group and clinical and academic staff put great energy and support into the implementation phase, the time after implementation is important for ensuring that all those involved in the new DEU understand and adhere to the model's key principles and indicators.

It is essential that staff understand their role in relation to the teaching and learning needs of students in their DEU and be willing to receive constructive feedback from the Working Group. Challenges encountered during the implementation phase include blurring of the CLN and/or ALN roles, tendency for the CLN to teach rather than facilitate student learning opportunities, the student assessment process not being completed collaboratively and managing geographically separate areas of the same DEU.

Moving a New DEU from the 'Initial' to the 'Established' Phase

We have found the implementation phase is crucial for ensuring that the key principles and indicators of the DEU model are understood and adhered to by all those involved in the new DEU. Anecdotal evidence from our Australian colleagues suggests that it takes about three semesters for the DEU model to become firmly embedded in a clinical area. Accordingly, the Working Group works closely with new DEU staff during the first three semesters to ensure that the key indicators of the DEU model are in place in preparation for moving into the established phase.

After an initial semester operating as a DEU, the following two semesters are termed the 'in maintenance' phase. During this time the area moves from preceptorship to a DEU way of operating. Having successfully implemented the DEU model, the DEU is considered to be established.

An established DEU has embraced the key principles of the DEU model and is able to function relatively independently of the Working Group. This decreases the workload for members of the Working Group and ensures that the ongoing maintenance of the DEU model remains manageable in the short term and sustainable over time.

The following criteria are used for identifying that a DEU model has been established:

- A minimum of three semesters using the DEU model of clinical teaching and learning have been completed.
- The education provider has appointed an ALN to the DEU and supports their attendance at annual DEU workshops and participation in evaluation meetings.
- The DEU's Charge Nurse Manager takes responsibility for 'appointing' an RN to the Clinical Liaison Role (CLN), ensuring the Checklist is completed for new CLN(s). The role is supported by rostering time for preparation, orientation and assessment; annual attendance at the DEU workshop; and attendance at CPIT's 'Introduction to Clinical Teaching Course for Registered Nurses'. All staff members receive DEU information in their orientation programme, and all nursing staff attend the CDHB Preceptor Level 1 and Level 2 courses. The CDHB Nurse Educator DEU is notified of CLN resignations and new appointments to key positions. Staff participation in evaluation meetings is encouraged.

Evaluation

Separate face-to-face evaluation meetings are held for DEU staff and students at the end of the first and third semester of working with the DEU model. The Working Group presents the summarised feedback from these meetings in a Summation Report to the Governance Group, with a recommendation that the DEU practice area move into the 'established' phase if all criteria are met. Once agreed, a letter is sent to the DEU practice area CNM, their direct line manager and the Director of Nursing, informing them that the practice area is now an 'Established DEU Practice Area' and providing an outline of what this means for the practice area and the organisation. A certificate (see example Fig. 11.11 in Edgecombe et al., Chap. 11, this volume) is presented to the practice area, clearly identifying its work with students using the DEU model of clinical teaching and learning. Each DEU is included in the ongoing audit process of the DEU model.

If results of the evaluation meeting indicate that the DEU practice area does not meet the criteria for moving into the established phase, the Working Group presents this finding to the Governance Group and puts in place supports including:

- DEU Working Group member(s) meet with the CNM, CLN and ALN to discuss the evaluation meeting results, identifying areas that need increased supports and implementing an action plan to address areas of concern.
- An evaluation meeting for staff and students at the end of the following semester using DEU key indicators.

If ongoing auditing reveals the DEU practice area is not meeting criteria for the established phase, or the CLN, DEU practice area or health organisation request help, the above supports are implemented. The DEU Working Group is available for ongoing support and assistance as needed.

Ongoing Audit and Evaluation

The Working Group is responsible for managing the workload associated with the ongoing maintenance of the DEU practice areas. Maintenance begins after the initial implementation phase and continues until the established phase and to a lesser extent after the requirements of the established phase are met. Once a DEU has become established, it goes onto a 2-yearly audit cycle. Separate evaluation processes have been developed for students and DEU staff. Each evaluation is facilitated by a Working Group member who is not directly involved with that particular group. The NE DEU and the Working Group collate the information and present it to staff, identifying what is working well, what needs attention and lessons learnt.

In response to the increasing numbers of DEUs, the Working Group is developing an online feedback tool for DEU staff. An online survey—the Clinical Learning Environment, Supervision and Nurse Teacher Scale (CLES+T) (Watson et al. 2010)—will be used to gather feedback from students at the end of their clinical placement. The survey contains 34 statements related to aspects of the clinical learning environment which address the themes of connecting with a community of clinical practice, role of the nurse teacher, supervisory relationship and learning opportunities. Reports can be provided to senior nurses from the clinical areas including DEUs, clinical lecturers and other teaching staff in a timely, useful and cost-effective manner.

Maintaining Quality

The Canterbury DEU model of clinical teaching and learning has been established for 3 years and will be reviewed 5 yearly. Whilst not all areas are able to use the DEU model, many are finding it effective for managing undergraduate nursing students undertaking clinical placements. Initial planning indicated the School of Nursing would require approximately 20 DEUs in 5 years, however, due to increasing student numbers and practice areas keen to become DEUs, we have 23 after 4 years. The ongoing management of new and established DEUs remains a challenge for the Working Group as most of the members have other key roles to perform for their respective organisations. The allocation of hours to the NE DEU role has helped to provide consistency and continuity with the ongoing DEU workload on a week-by-week basis whilst allowing members of the Working Group to juggle their time and commitments and still actively contribute to the DEU model. Strategies implemented to maintain quality in DEUs were:

Face-to-face evaluation meetings
DEU key indicators
Audit planner
Review of DEU documents (includes philosophy, roles and responsibilities)
Annual DEU Workshop
Providing support to existing DEUs (includes updating intranet and Internet)
Ongoing promotion of the model (includes updating information brochure and website)
Ongoing maintenance of the model
Support from DEU Governance Group

Future Directions

Canterbury was the first region in New Zealand to use the DEU model of clinical teaching and learning. The level of interest generated by the DEU project was not anticipated. We assisted a community nursing provider to set up a Community DEU (Betony and Yarwood 2010) and started another one in 2011. We have hosted many visitors from District Health Boards and educational institutes who are interested in setting up DEUs in partnership. Visitors gain clarity about how a DEU works by talking to key staff in several DEUs, and the Working Group share experiences and resources.

An Internet page has been developed to provide DEU staff with access to information about key roles, student courses, staff and student responsibilities, and how to contact members of the Working Group. Frequently asked questions are included, and all the DEU documents are available. A DVD gives an overview of the DEU, the key roles, benefits for staff and students and how to find out more.

The DVD can be viewed online via the DEU website http://www.cdhb.govt.nz/deu/default.htm.

The development of closer collaboration between CPIT, CDHB and the Canterbury Health System has strengthened relationships. A 5-year strategic plan is being developed, encompassing joint research and quality projects. Initial discussions have been held regarding students' transition to practice following their final placement in a DEU, how they might move into new graduate positions within a DEU and how other new graduate nurses may be supported by this model.

The DEU model offers students the opportunity to practise direction and delegation skills in the 'real world', as 1st, 2nd and 3rd year students are on placement in a DEU at the same time. Another opportunity for this is emerging with the introduction of the Diploma in Enrolled Nursing, which commenced in New Zealand in 2011. The Working Group's plans for 2011 included working with another District Health Board on the implementation of DEUs.

Conclusion

In Canterbury, the DEU model has strengthened partnerships between the education provider and the clinical practice areas. This has permeated through all levels starting with the nurse leaders of CPIT and CDHB, down to the successful partnerships between the ALNs and the CLNs. The successful partnership between the DEU Working Group members has also ensured that the DEU model has moved forward. Resources from the CPIT/CDHB model are used in Edgecombe et al. (Chap. 11, this volume) as examples of how to do a DEU.

Whilst nursing has driven the implementation of DEUs, this model of supporting undergraduate students' clinical learning has much to offer all health professional students. There is potential for it to become an interprofessional DEU, a direction requiring research, new collaborative partnerships and piloting. The University of Portland, Oregon's newest DEU model that involves nursing students working as part of an interprofessional care team (Craig and Moscato, Chap. 6, this volume) highlights the possibilities for interprofessional DEUs.

Acknowledgement Michelle, Deb and Jane wish to acknowledge the support of Isabel Jamieson, Rose Whittle, Raylene Shaw, Debbie Cook and Teresa Kilkenny in this endeavour.

References

Betony, K., & Yarwood, J. (2010). Adapting the Dedicated Education Unit model for student learning in the community. *Kai Tiaki Nursing New Zealand, 16*(5), 22–23.

Budgen, C., & Gamroth, L. (2008). An overview of practice education models. *Nurse Education Today, 28*(3), 273–283.

Cardno, C. (2003). *Action research: A developmental approach*. Wellington: New Zealand Council for Educational Research.

Cardno, C., & Piggot-Irvine, E. (1994, November). *Action research—The key to successful senior management training in schools*. In Proceedings of the NZARE conference. NZARE, Christchurch, New Zealand.

Casey, M., Jamieson, I., Hale, J., Sims, D., Whittle, R., & Kilkenny, T. (2008). Dedicated Education Units—A new way of supporting clinical learning. *Kai Tiaki Nursing New Zealand, 14*(11), 24–25.

Crawford, M., & Whittle, R. (2008, September). *Supporting clinical learning. Clinical leadership: Supporting DEUs*. Presentation, 13th National Nurse Educators Conference, Sydney, Australia.

Hale, J., & Jamieson, I. (2009, September 30–October 2). *Dedicated Education Units: Enhancing nurse students' belongingness*. Power point presentation at 'Working together: Education and practice'. Australasian Nurse Educators Conference, Christchurch, New Zealand.

IBM software. (n.d.). *SPSS*. http://www-01.ibm.com/software/analytics/spss/

Jamieson, I., Hale, J., Sims, D., Casey, M., Whittle, R., & Kilkenny, T. (2008). *Establishing Dedicated Education Units for undergraduate nursing students: Pilot project summation report*. Christchurch: CPIT.

KPMG. (2001). *Strategic review of undergraduate nursing education: Report to Nursing Council of New Zealand*. Resource document. Wellington: Nursing Council of New Zealand. http://www.nursingcouncil.org.nz/download/48/kpmg-strategic-review.pdf. Accessed 11 Oct 2010.

Levett-Jones, T., & Lathlean, J. (2008). Belongingness: A prerequisite for nursing students' clinical learning. *Nurse Education in Practice, 8*(2), 103–111.

Levett-Jones, T., Lathlean, J., Higgins, I., & McMillan, M. (2009). Staff and student relationships and their impact on nursing students' belongingness and learning. *Journal of Advanced Nursing, 65*(2), 316–324.

Street, A. F. (2004). Action research. In V. Minichiello, G. Sullivan, K. Greenwood, & S. R. Axford (Eds.), *The handbook of research methods for nursing and health science* (2nd ed.). Sydney: Prentice Hall Health.

Watson, P., Seaton, P., Sims, D., Jamieson, I., Whittle, R., & Saarikoski, M. (2010). *Evaluating the quality of workplace learning for student nurses in hospital settings*. Christchurch: CPIT & Ako Aotearoa.

Chapter 8
Dedicated Educational Unit: A Scandinavian Model

Margaretha Ekebergh

> *Glossary of Terms in Order of Appearance in This Chapter*
>
> Primary Tutor Register ed Nurse (RN) or certified nursing assistant who guides students in concrete care and learning situations
>
> Secondary Tutor Registered Nurse (RN) or certified nursing assistant who guides students in concrete care and learning situations
>
> Teacher an academic from the University who bridges theory and best practice in the students' clinical education

Introduction

The Dedicated Educational Unit (DEU) from a Swedish perspective is a learning environment where caring and learning are united in what we call 'reflective tutoring'. The overall purpose of the DEU is to support the nursing students' learning process in terms of integrating theory with best practice and their professional development. On a research basis, the DEU has been implemented in medical, orthopaedic, rehabilitation, geriatric and psychiatric care as well as in municipal health care. A DEU treats 15–24 patients at a time (this varies with the different DEUs) and hosts approximately 12 students during their clinicalstudies. The students'

M. Ekebergh (✉)
School of Health Sciences, Borås University, Borås, Sweden
e-mail: margaretha.ekebergh@hb.se

K. Edgecombe and M. Bowden (eds.), *Clinical Learning and Teaching Innovations in Nursing*, Innovation and Change in Professional Education 10,
DOI 10.1007/978-94-007-7232-8_8, © Springer Science+Business Media Dordrecht 2014

learning is patient centred, which means that students maintain continuity in their patient relations during their clinical studies. This is organised in such a way that each student is associated with one or several patients and is tutored by the nurses and nursing assistants in charge. The idea is that the student progressively takes responsibility for these patients' care. The degree and extent of student responsibility is dependent on the student's educational level. Such patient-centred learning does not mean that the student has one personal tutor but that a primary tutor is responsible for the continuity of conducting the tutoring. This manner of organising tutorship has proved successful for enhancing the students' prerequisites for independence and taking on responsibility in their learning processes (Ekebergh and Määttä 2005). Not only do the students increase their knowledge and deepen their understanding of a patient's entire situation, but their critical reflection is also promoted in terms of approach, values, abilities and conception of care work. The students are forced to rethink and compare alternative actions in order to form an opinion of different approaches and caring actions (Ekebergh and Määttä 2005).

Key Tutoring Roles

A tutoring team in a Borås University DEU consists of primary tutors, secondary tutors and a teacher. Their roles are briefly summarised as:

Primary tutors are Registered Nurses (RNs) with specific competence in the main field of nurse education (caring science) as well as in didactics and tutoring. The primary tutor has the overall responsibility for conducting the students' clinical studies. Each DEU has 1–2 primary tutors.

Secondary tutors are Registered Nurses (RNs) who guide the students in concrete care and learning situations. This role could also be played by a certified nursing assistant during certain fundamental care procedures. A DEU is comprised of nurses and nursing assistants with an interest in tutoring and developing care.

A teacher is an academic from the educational institution who bridges theory and best practice in the students' clinical education (Lindahl et al. 2009).

Foundational Premises of the Borås University DEUs

A DEU is formed and established based on the following premises:

1. Scientific basis (based in Caring Science)
2. Reflective approach
3. The lifeworld perspective as a reference frame for learning and tutoring
4. Clear strategies for caring and learning as parallel and common phenomena
5. Qualified tutoring
6. Clear learning progression

7. Active patient care development
8. Focus on the research team's possibilities in care work and learning

These premises are explained in the next part of this chapter.

A Scientific Basis

A DEU is based on caring science[1] in which knowledge may enable deeper understanding for the patient and his/her situation in terms of health and suffering, with the purpose of providing optimal care. A holistic view is central in caring science, which means that the patient is always given attention and is understood from his/her context. The patient cannot be separated from his/her lived world and all it contains. The patient's perspective can be ascribed a deeper understanding by use of caring science definitions such as the 'lifeworld', 'suffering', 'wellbeing/health', 'subjective lived body' and 'caring relation' (Dahlberg et al. 2003). The patient perspective is characterised by an ethical approach signified by respect, integrity and dignity. This is concretised in the caring sector in that care must have its starting point in the patient's story.

In a DEU, the patient perspective is key; it is the perspective from which care work is organised and conducted. In practice, this concerns routines, general care plans and quality enhancement work to be reviewed and assessed in relation to the patient's perspective. The caring science knowledge comprises the main field of nurse education: it is the knowledge the students must acquire and apply in patient-close practice. This is why there needs to be congruence between theory and best practice in a DEU. All learning must start from the entirety, which would be the patient's story, because caring science is a holistic perspective. Using the patient's story as the starting point, knowledge from disciplines such as medicine, caring science and psychology are interwoven into the learning process.

Reflective Approach

A DEU has pronounced awareness of the importance of reflection for students' learning as well as caregivers' development and growth. In order to develop and deepen the understanding of what reflection is in relation to learning and caring, continuous education concerning both the epistemology of reflection and its practice is necessary for caregivers. Reflective practice is rooted in lifeworld theory (Husserl 1973, 1998). It takes place both when meeting with the patient and when intertwining theory with best practice during group or individual tutoring. Again

[1]Caring science is the main field of nurse education and the subject in which the students are awarded their academic bachelor's degree.

I emphasise that reflection is key; it must always be related to knowledge in caring science and lifeworld perspectives. Different forms of reflection used in tutorship should be assessed and problematised on this basis instead of being viewed as a separate method or technique (Ekebergh 2007).

A scientific basis may be developed through reflection. This is a central purpose of studying in a DEU. The students learn to systematically problematise and reflect on issues, draw conclusions, assess and document knowledge based on concrete clinical practices (Lindahl et al. 2009).

The Lifeworld Perspective as a Reference Frame for Learning and Tutoring

In a DEU, the lifeworld perspective is the fundamental approach to learning. This means that the learner's world of experiences (i.e. the lifeworld) is the starting point for all learning support. Learning is individual and takes its point of departure from the learner's previous experiences, which accompany the learning process. Each individual has a specific learning profile depending on one's subjective dimension in terms of understanding, values, interests and perspectives. This demands an open approach when meeting the learner, both in individual and group tutoring as well as during practical studies, when planning tutoring sessions and when assessing the learner's achievements. Concretely, in a DEU, one's openness to the learner's experiences and subjectivity is expressed in individual study plans. The lifeworld perspective does not accept general study plans or rigid tutoring methods (Ekebergh 2005).

The students in a DEU are to acquire knowledge and competence by use of various forms of education, for example theme seminars, individual tutoring, reflective group tutoring sessions or other forms of reflection, group work with care problems and training in different practical skills. DEU studies include theoretical studies as well as the experience-based knowledge that develops when students participate in and take responsibility for patients' care. Experiences and care actions must be followed by reflection and assessment to achieve optimal learning because experiences and actions per se do not automatically result in new knowledge and understanding. They require conscious processing and reviewing to qualify as new knowledge and insights. Emotions and conceptions are clarified when an experience is expressed in words.

The students are trained to verbally communicate their thoughts and emotions with their tutor or tutoring group, which enables the development of a reflective approach. Experiences from care work are given a deeper significance by use of definitions relevant to caring science. Then, the student learns how such definitions can be used as tools to increase understanding of a patient's situation and needs, as well as for care itself. At the same time, theoretical concepts are brought to life when applied in concrete care situations. Theoretical knowledge and best practice are intertwined in the learning process, strengthened by the caring science reflective group tutoring sessions.

Clear Strategies for Caring and Learning as Parallel and Common Phenomena

In a DEU, learning and caring go hand in hand; neither has precedence over the other. From a lifeworld perspective, learning and caring have the same characteristics. The caring science perspective—interest in the patient and his/her world—is a fundamental trait expressed in the learning context, where interest is directed towards learning in a similar way as in the caring context. Thus, the caring and the learning relations are alike in terms of showing respect, creating a sense of security, showing trust and being supportive. What promotes learning also promotes caring and vice versa, which is why this approach leads to developing and creating good care. If there is an apparent consistency between caring and learning (i.e. message and action overlap), students learn in greater depth about what caring is. This demands a tutor who is sensitive and responsive to the students' learning needs as well as attentive to the patients' care needs. Therefore, the tutor needs an integrated perspective on caring science and must have 'lived' what he/she teaches. In this way, the caring science perspective is woven into the tutoring sessions so that scientific theories are tied to concrete reality. Symbolically, 'head, hand and heart' are important parts of the tutor's approach.

In a concrete sense, this perspective of the connection between caring and learning is expressed in the planning of all care work; the planned learning is considered and vice versa. The DEU challenge is to develop strategies that affirm and clarify the fundamental principle that caring and learning are parallel and common phenomena in order to better support and develop the patients' care.

Qualified Tutoring

In a DEU, all staff have fundamental knowledge in tutoring as well as in caring science. In the tutoring team, with its primary and secondary tutors and clinical teachers, the teachers hold overall responsibility for didactic issues and initiate tutoring strategies to adequately combine theory and best practice. DEU tutors gain their experiences from being tutors, but they also need support for growing and developing their tutorship. Here, the clinical teachers play an important part as they guide the secondary tutors in tutorship individually as well as in groups. Also, the primary tutor needs guidance in providing learning support and integrating theory with clinical practice. This should be organised in groups where a clinical senior lecturer or lecturer leads the primary tutor. The clinical teachers also conduct group tutoring sessions and other suitable tutorship with the students together with the primary and secondary tutors. The primary tutor holds higher competence in tutoring as well as in the subject (a Master's degree in caring science) and thereby not only leads the learning work at the DEU but also functions as a significant resource for the secondary tutors. Clinical senior lecturers are scientific and pedagogical resources for the DEU as they work closely with the clinical lecturers and lead specialised activities in the subject and in didactics.

Clear Learning Progression

Learning progression is an important part of a DEU. Each DEU has a certain educational level (some may have two) in relation to the education programme as a whole. The level for each DEU should have a pronounced awareness of the students' learning processes during their clinical studies and should relate this to their individual study plans. The DEU should take an active lead in developing and creating structures and other strategies to ensure that the learning progression is in line with the lifeworld perspective as a basis for learning.

Active Patient Care Development

A DEU has favourable conditions for the natural integration of research and development projects. The aim is to have continuously running projects that include students, tutors, teachers and researchers. Strategies for starting this activity are currently under way. The research projects ought to be large scale so that their parts can be distributed to different DEUs depending on the project's character and research questions. The clinical lecturers play an important part in conducting the projects, as well as creating conditions for their commencement. Other scientific competence may be brought in depending on the project's character. What is of the utmost importance here is a united front so that all students, teachers, researchers and practitioners involved in the project strive towards the same goal—research-based care and a learning environment. It is also important to produce high quality research, which should be possible with interdisciplinary and interprofessional projects. One extensive research programme on integrated care development, which will be conducted partly in a DEU, is currently under development.

Focus on Possibilities for the Research Team in Care Work and Learning

In a DEU, the patient perspective is key, which implicitly means having an interest in how different care competences and professions work together for giving patients optimal care from a holistic perspective. Having an interest in the patient perspective generates a different view from the traditional one in which each profession is separated from the whole in order to fulfil one's duty. Instead of this separation there is a pronounced desire to develop the team's possibilities for improved care; an idea for development in the DEU in the future. Pilot projects can include interventions that aim to develop strategies for team work, which has a thorough foundation and a core characterised by innovation. The team also becomes central for learning support, which should enrich, broaden and deepen understandings of the patient and different caring actions.

Results of Research into the DEU's Effectiveness as a Clinical Learning Environment: Informing Future Development

The potential and deficits of tutoring emerged in an interview study with a phenomenological analysis of how DEU tutoring supports students' learning (Ekebergh and Määttä 2005). Results are summarised here into six themes that characterise a DEU as seen from the students' and tutors' perspectives:

- Individualised didactics
- Learning environment
- Patient-centred learning
- Place for reflection
- Caring science in practice
- A unit with pedagogic potential

According to the results, successful tutorship takes its point of departure from the student and his/her lifeworld. The didactics in the DEU creates a learning atmosphere characterised by the premise that every student is understood as a unique learning individual with a specific learning profile.

Results show that the tutoring situation constitutes the area for the meeting between theoretical and general caring science, and concrete, lived experiences in patient-close contexts. The essence of knowledge constituted by the patients' lived experiences of illness, disease and suffering feels close and real to the students. Therefore, the students' reflections have their starting points in the patients' lifeworlds. However, during the reflection process, the students need support to integrate lived experiences with theoretical knowledge in order to gain a deeper or newer understanding of the caring phenomena related to the patient's world. In the ideal tutoring situation, where the tutor is well acquainted with the essence of knowledge both in theory and in practice, this process promotes development of the student's knowledge and understanding.

The research has identified that the DEU contains rich possibilities for concretising caring theory into practice. Students who have acquired and understood the meaning of theoretical caring science and have developed a reflective approach can grasp the patient perspective as the main focus and draw attention to it during care. Students discover and understand patterns of complexity of the patients' perspectives through 'conscious reflection', which is an embodied learning process that incorporates thought, emotion and action in both theory and best practice.

Conclusion and Future Prospects

In order to grow a beneficial learning environment in a DEU, good soil is needed. This soil is composed of people with a strong interest in cultivation and a genuine will to create optimal conditions for integrating caring theory with best practice and the art of care. Secondary tutors with 'green fingers' contribute to this process. However, the managers, primary tutors and clinical teachers are the key persons for promoting growth in the learning environment. The clinical teachers fulfil a special function by providing nutrition to the cultivation through their mission to bridge the gap between theory and best practice. Therefore, it is of the utmost importance for the future cultivation of the DEU that competences in tutoring and reflection are further developed and deepened for the tutoring teams (the primary and secondary tutors and clinical teachers). This will ensure that the good soil is preserved and nurtured so that research results can provide even better support for learning.

References

Dahlberg, K., Segesten, K., Nyström, M., Suserud, B-O., & Fagerberg, I. (2003). *Att förstå vårdvetenskap* [Understanding caring science]. Lund: Studentlitteratur.

Ekebergh, M. (2005). Are you in control of the method or is the method in control of you? *Nurse Educator, 30*(6), 259–262.

Ekebergh, M. (2007). Lifeworld-based reflection and learning: A contribution to the reflective practice in nursing and nursing education. *Reflective Practice, 8*(3), 331–343.

Ekebergh, M., & Määttä, S. (2005). *Lärandet på en utbildningsvårdsavdelning—att sammanbinda vårdvetenskaplig teori med vårdpraxis* [Learning in an Educational Unit—intertwining caring science in theory with caring practices]. Forskningsrapport, Institutionen för Vårdvetenskap, Högskolan i Borås Rapport nr 1 (Research report). Borås: School of Health Care Sciences, Borås University.

Husserl, E. (1973). *Experience and judgment.* Evanston: North Western University Press.

Husserl, E. (1998). *Ideas pertaining to a pure phenomenology and a phenomenological philosophy* (F. Kersten, Trans.). Dordrecht: Kluwer Academic.

Lindahl, B., Dagborn, K., & Nilsson, M. (2009). A student-centred Clinical Education Unit—description of a reflective learning model. *Nurse Education in Practice, 9*(1), 5–12.

Chapter 9
Building Clinical and Academic Staff and Student Capacity in Dedicated Education Units

Kay Edgecombe and Margaret Bowden

Glossary of Terms in Order of Appearance in This Chapter

Capacity building   professional staff and student development/preparation for DEU teaching roles

ANMC Competencies   Australian Nursing and Midwifery Council competencies required for registration as a nurse (RN) or midwife (RM) (ANMC n.d.)

Principal Academic (PA)   an academic lecturer in clinical (nursing school faculty member) who visits the clinical setting prior to student placement to facilitate clinical staff preparation for working with the students and thereafter visits the clinical setting regularly throughout each semester; communicates and liaises with students, the LN and the CNC, and utilises their ongoing expertise to facilitate students' learning

Dedicated Liaison Nurse (DLN)/Clinical Liaison Nurse (CLN)   an experienced Registered Nurse (RN) selected from the practice area who takes on extra responsibilities, including overseeing clinical learning in the DEU and liaising between staff, students and academics/faculty the liaison between the unit and the University Academic Liaison Nurse (ALN) a permanent clinical lecturer at the University who provides consistent support to students and clinicians

K. Edgecombe (✉) • M. Bowden
School of Nursing and Midwifery, Flinders University, GPO Box 2100,
Adelaide, South Australia, Australia, 5001
e-mail: kay.edgecombe@flinders.edu.au; margaret.bowden@internode.on.net;
margaret.bowden@flinders.edu.au

K. Edgecombe and M. Bowden (eds.), *Clinical Learning and Teaching Innovations in Nursing*, Innovation and Change in Professional Education 10,
DOI 10.1007/978-94-007-7232-8_9, © Springer Science+Business Media Dordrecht 2014

Registered Nurse (RN) College- or University-qualified nurse licensed by a nursing registration body to undertake all facets of nursing in accordance with the body's regulations

Enrolled Nurse (EN) Diploma-qualified nurse working under supervision of a RN to provide nursing care

Clinical Instructor (CI) a staff nurse who wants to teach

Clinical Faculty Coordinator (CFC) nursing faculty from the University who plans students' experience and informs Clinical Instructors (CI) what is covered in University classes each week

Introduction

The Dedicated Education Unit (DEU) is a set of principles and concepts that enable change in curriculum and clinical learning contexts while maintaining increased student time and opportunity for clinical learning throughout their journey to becoming professional nurses. DEUs are designed to encompass clinical and academic staff capacity building through designating DEU-specific roles and responsibilities, such as Liaison Nurse/Dedicated Liaison Nurse (LN/DLN), Clinical Nurse Consultant (CNC) or Principal Academic (PA), as described in Chaps. 2, 4, 5, 6, 7, 8, 10 and 11 (this volume). The basic design whereby clinical staff act as nursing students' primary clinical instructors in the clinical setting generates clinical staff capacity building as they go about their day-to-day work with students in the DEU (see Craig and Moscato, Chap. 6, this volume). However, it is still essential to provide clinical staff with enhanced opportunities to learn how to teach students, as recommended by Benner et al. (2010), in the interests of improved nursing education and patient safety.

It is not only clinical staff who need these opportunities to learn how to teach nursing students. Academic staff benefit by maintaining the currency of their clinical knowledge and skills to inform their classroom teaching. Students develop further educative skills in the DEU context of peer teaching and learning. Curriculum and assessment are key considerations when designing formal capacity building strategies/events, considerations based on the fact that patient safety is paramount. Reshaping the timing of clinical placements to privilege clinical equally with the theory of classroom work (Bail et al., Chap. 5, this volume) as a curriculum design strategy, for example, engenders greater integration of the two, and greater sharing and valuing of clinician and academic knowledge, thus supporting capacity building for all DEU staff.

Capacity Building and Curriculum: The Influence of Learning Outcomes, Graduate Attributes and Competencies

Achieving the formal and incidental learning outcomes, reflected in graduate attributes and nursing competencies relevant to the country in which a DEU is operating, is a goal for which students, clinicians and academics strive. In the DEU, the outcomes surpass the designated learning objectives. There is a need to build student, clinician and academic capacity in DEUs to ensure they meet the goals. The original Flinders University School of Nursing philosophy statements reflect the need to design the curriculum to take account of two potentially conflicting goals in nurse education: to prepare students 'for beginning level practice as registered nurses ... [and] to develop cognitive skills, values and attitudes which will prepare them for lifelong learning and reflective practice' (FUSON 1991: 20). Curriculum design, including peer teaching and learning in DEUs, and other ways of engaging students as partners with academics and clinical staff in learning theory and practice, such as student feedback sessions, have a direct influence on students' achievement of their goals. The value of student feedback sessions is evidenced in a statement by DEU students Anj Taylor and Vandhana Nand (Story 1, Chap. 10, this volume): 'We've changed a lot already through the feedback sessions and these changes have been put in place for the next DEU. We feel so valued; our voices were heard'.

Capacity Building in Assessment and Feedback

As identified by Grealish et al. (Chap. 3, this volume), the area of clinical assessment remains a challenging component of nursing education for clinicians and academics (Cowan et al. 2005; McAllister 1998). The never-ending question of how to assess the student's progress towards becoming a competent novice RN leads to a critical focus on forms of assessment and who is best placed to undertake them. Therefore, much capacity building for DEU clinical and academic staff has an assessment focus. The argument is put forward in Taylor and Nand (Story 1, Chap. 10, this volume) that 'assessments are harder in DEUs because the tutors are there all the time. With other students, assessment is just a process. It is not going on all the time'.

Clinicians and academics need to be equipped with the capacity to understand and acknowledge the possibility that the different biases of employer expectations and academic expectations can influence the way students are assessed. Clinical facilitators (academics) assess students as beginning practitioners, whereas clinicians may assess students from a workplace perspective—how ready students are to start work—rather than from the perspective of students as learners.

Building Capacity in the Language of Assessment

The language of assessment is explained in formal capacity building strategies such as workshops. This language must reflect the clinical learning environment—learning assessment tools (competencies)—and this language is not common to nurses' clinical situation. Therefore, it is necessary to build clinicians' capacity to have a greater understanding of the meaning of academic language and to modify the assessment criteria/language to better reflect the clinical learning environment meaning and context. For example, a highly experienced nurse, using the intuitive knowledge that comes with their experience, might say to a clinical facilitator, 'That student will make a good nurse', or 'That student is going to fail'. Capacity building involves giving clinical staff a language to describe this and to use the language in an informed way. Developing the language of assessment in clinicians may be as simple as asking for specific details such as time, place, what, when and how when someone says, 'This student has a problem'. When someone says, 'This student is achieving well', they need to give a specific description, for example, 'The Student looked after x patient and was able to . . . ' (specific details of what they did well and how they did it well, 'They did this, this and this'). Then the nurse needs to identify what difference the student has made to the patient outcome or the clinicians' outcomes. This detail is needed when assessing students in terms of registration board competencies.

Understanding and practising the language of assessment helps clinicians and academics validate their assessments. It gives them the language needed to stand up in front of their colleagues and validate what might otherwise seem to be nuanced assessment, a subjective judgement based solely on the assessor's level of practice expertise (Benner 1984), without objective explanation. The language also enables clinicians and academics to identify and talk about the biases and noise (e.g. culture and other distractions from the objectives of the assessment) that might impact their assessment. It enables them to identify the criteria for accountability of their assessment as a way of evaluating the effectiveness of the approaches to teaching and learning in different clinical contexts. Particularly important in capacity building for DEU staff is assisting them to assess in a progressive manner because students are in the unit over an extended time. The different structure of DEUs requires assessors to validate specific concepts being addressed over time. For example, when they see a student doing something, assessors need to look back to what the student did previously, rather than simply assessing the students' current performance. Looking back to the student's previous performance is an important step in establishing rigour in the assessment process and evaluating the student's progression in both their learning and labour force practice.

Building Capacity in Understanding Different Types of Assessment

Understanding the different types of assessment and their benefit or limitations is also a necessary part of capacity building for staff and students in DEUs. Therefore, sessions are needed for clinicians, academics and students on understanding formative, summative and self-assessment. In the DEU, constructive ongoing feedback and constant assessment add rigour to the whole assessment process. 'Assessors (clinicians) are right there all the time with the students' (Taylor and Nand, Story 1, Chap. 10, this volume); they become familiar with the students so they can observe progressions or regressions and effectively intervene to optimise students' progress or step in to address any problems. Students' learning is not limited—students progressing well can be given increased opportunity for autonomy, while those requiring greater support have the support on hand. Peer teaching plays an important role in students being able to facilitate each other's learning, assess each other's progress and audit self-assessments.

As described by Bail et al. (Chap. 5, this volume), students are supported to self-assess as a component of their formative assessment part way through their placement. Students are provided with the *ANMC Competencies* (ANMC n.d.) (utilised for registration of nurses in Australia) and asked to describe examples where they have demonstrated components of nursing practice, such as 'practices within an ethical nursing framework' or 'establishes and maintains therapeutic relationships'. The students self-assess performance against the standards, utilising the Bondy Rating Scale (1983).

Formative assessment is provided informally in meetings with the Principal Academic (PA) and/or the Dedicated Liaison Nurse (DLN) and includes discussion, feedback and feedforward. The PA and/or the DLN conduct summative feedback, which is part of the final assessment. This is again graded against the *ANMC Competencies* (ANMC n.d.) using the Bondy Rating Scale. The final assessment takes place at a meeting with the student and is based on three major sources of evidence: student self-assessment, PA judgement on attitudes and knowledge based on critical conversations over the semester, and specific feedback about clinical skills and attitudes from clinicians with whom the students have worked. This ongoing summative assessment contributes to progressive learning across placements throughout the students' degree. The meeting also has a formative aspect, and students are encouraged to identify their learning needs for the next months of their careers. The ongoing and collaborative nature of assessment acts as a capacity building tool, enabling clinicians, academics (clinical facilitators) and students to learn to assess through practice.

In the Canterbury, New Zealand, DEU model described in Chap. 7, the Clinical Liaison Nurse (CLN) and Academic Liaison Nurse (ALN) undertake students' formative and summative assessments. They introduced this process to promote the role of the DEU staff as clinical teachers and to provide a consistent and valid assessment process because students work with multiple nurses. The student completes their self-assessment and gives it to the CLN or ALN the day prior to assessment. The ALN and CLN discuss the student's self-assessment and their own estimation of the student's progress, after which the student joins the meeting to discuss their progress and set goals for the remainder of the placement. Summative assessments follow a similar format. Thus, the way assessment is undertaken is a capacity building strategy.

In the Swedish DEU (Ekebergh, Chap. 8, this volume), emphasis is placed on learning progression. Each DEU has a certain educational level (some may have two) in relation to the education programme as a whole. The level for each DEU should have a pronounced awareness of the students' learning processes during their clinical studies and should relate this to their individual study plans. The DEU should take an active lead in developing and creating structures and other strategies to ensure that the learning progression is in line with the lifeworld perspective as a basis for learning.

Capacity Building for Feedback in the Clinical Setting

Clinicians, academics and students need capacity building for feedback processes in clinical settings. Feedback is very contextual and more immediate than assessment, spanning complex or simplistic and linear experiences. As Bail et al. explain in Chap. 5 (this volume), the restructured Canberra University nursing curriculum placed added emphasis on the feedback students gain in both clinical and theoretical components of their learning and how it 'feeds forward' to affect their professional development. Feedback contains the crucial 'sandwich component', telling the student what they've done well, where they can improve and giving them some insight into how they can improve. This component is also about assessment.

Workshops, as described in the next section, are key structured events for building the capacity of clinical and academic staff in DEUs. Preliminary face-to-face preparation sessions for DEU students detailing peer teaching and learning are a strategy used to build students' capacity for self- and peer assessment as part of overall preparation for learning and working in the clinical context.

Formal Capacity Building Strategies for DEU Clinical and Academic Staff

Formal, structured, scheduled activities designed to build DEU staff capacity include clinical staff completing clinical feedback forms and evaluation surveys; involving clinical staff in student orientation to DEUs; involving academics and students in ward team meetings; academic and clinical staff liaison regarding student behaviour and performance; and inviting clinical and academic staff to become members of a practice development working party (Bail et al., Chap. 5, this volume). However, workshops have become the most common form of structured capacity building for clinical and academic DEU staff (Gonda, Chap. 4, Bail et al., Chap. 5 and Casey et al., Chap. 7, this volume). They have been proven successful as capacity building strategies.

Workshops

Workshops, held predominantly at Universities but sometimes in clinical venues, are designed to help clinical staff understand what the students are learning in the classroom and what their expected learning objectives are at a particular year level. The formal and incidental learning outcomes are also explored in the context of specific DEUs. The workshops are also designed to help academics keep in touch with the latest changes in the clinical setting. They aim to develop clinicians' and academics' capacity to integrate the University and clinical curriculums, to share knowledge and experiences, develop firm relationships and be well prepared to teach and assess students in DEUs. One of the greatest benefits of holding workshops at the Universities is that clinical and academic staff from all DEUs can attend, whereas workshops held in a clinical venue only accommodate clinical and academic staff from that venue. For example, University of Canberra (UC) holds a 'Mega DEU' once a year. All Dedicated Liaison Nurses (DLN) and DEU clinical managers are invited to a forum as an opportunity to develop collaboratively and learn from each other. Clinicians working with health students on clinical placements provided by UC are also invited to twice-yearly free workshops (Bail et al., Chap. 5, this volume). In Canterbury, New Zealand, CPIT/CDHB runs workshops each semester to educate clinical and academic staff undertaking key roles in the DEU for the first time, and to update existing DEU staff on curriculum changes and provide opportunities to problem solve issues and look for quality assurance and research opportunities (Casey et al., Chap. 7, this volume).

The original workshop concept resulted from staff feedback to the PAs after the Flinders University School of Nursing DEU pilot. It arose in response to expressions of interest and comments from DEU staff. One-day workshops were made available to all nursing staff (Registered Nurses-RNs and Enrolled Nurses-ENs) in the DEU. Workshops were offered strategically at the beginning of the year in the 2–3 weeks prior to clinical commencing to ensure workshop participants are still in the DEU when the students arrive. The workshops were also offered on 6 days to enable as many nursing staff as possible to attend on different days without disrupting the nursing rosters. Initially, staff members were seconded. The school paid this cost as well as catering costs; lunch, morning and afternoon tea provided irreplaceable networking opportunities for clinical and academic staff and a valuable extension of the whole workshop experience. These breaks were invaluable for both professional and personal networking and informal brainstorming of ideas about DEUs, how this one did it differently from that one, and shared support for concerns clinicians raised. The DEU venues considered the workshops to be a valuable professional development for their staff. Today it would count towards the 20 h mandatory professional development they are required to complete.

One significant DEU venue chose to have a workshop on their site as an alternative arrangement. This was carried out in order to meet the staff capacity building objective. However, having the workshops on-site minimised the opportunities for networking with DEU staff from other sites.

Whenever a new DEU was developed, maximum numbers of staff were encouraged to attend the workshops. Any new staff members in long-established DEUs were encouraged to attend. Clinical facilitators (PAs) employed by the University who would go to hand over time several times prior to the students' arrival in the DEU also attended the workshops.

A Flinders University School of Nursing one-day workshop programme is given here as an example of a clinical and academic staff capacity building opportunity.

1. *Meet and greet*. The workshop begins with a meet and greet, where clinical and academic staff can meet each other, identify which DEUs they are in, what their roles are and get an overview of different DEUs. This introductory time also enables staff to meet the course coordinators and clinical placement coordinators with whom they will be in contact.
2. *Overview of the DEU experience: the nature of the team*. After meeting and greeting, the DEU coordinator presents a brief overview of the DEU experience: the nature of the team. The coordinator explains the principles behind the DEU and how it came to be, then gives a brief presentation of how it works in the clinical setting. Workshop participants see a variety of DEU configurations (e.g. mental health, acute surgical) to demonstrate how the DEU adapts to the particular learning environment.
3. *Undergraduate nursing programme*. Course coordinators give a short presentation outlining the undergraduate nursing programme. This is essential to the clinicians' understanding of what students are learning across the entire programme; it gives a whole of the curriculum picture and helps build another bridge between the University and clinical learning contexts.
4. *Specific semester topics, clinical direction and assessment*. Topic coordinators give the final presentation before morning tea in which they explain specific semester topics and talk about clinical direction and assessment. Topics covered included facilitating theory to practice transfer of students' learning; fulfilling the topic objectives in the clinical setting; assessment details related to the clinical experience; and who is to do assessment (clinical staff or the PA). In the final semester, assessment is a formal process between the PA and a clinical staff member who is in a position to have informed input.
5. *Supporting clinical learning*. This session details teaching and learning strategies staff can use, including thinking aloud, small blocks of knowledge building into larger knowledge or having an umbrella to hook pieces of knowledge into relevant practice, situated learning, principles of reflection in practice, and peer learning and teaching—explaining the theory behind the clinicians' practice of teaching the students in clinical.
6. *Lunch.* personal and professional networking between work colleagues, previous clinical contacts and academics. This casual capacity building enables academics to catch up on what is happening regarding development and changes in clinical venues.
7. *Clinical coaching and the Liaison Nurse (LN) role.* A short presentation about clinical coaching and the Liaison Nurse (LN) role follows lunch. It focuses

on facilitating optimal learning outcomes for students by identifying their strengths, supporting ongoing development/identifying areas of concern and initiating appropriate interventions. One intervention DEU clinical and academic staff need to understand is the clinical learning contract; a contract designed to provide students at risk of failing the clinical component of a nursing practice topic with the opportunity to focus on areas of unsatisfactory practice identified by clinical staff. Students work collaboratively with clinical coaches and PAs to successfully complete the contract and the clinical component of their course. The contract consists of clearly stated clinical practice issues that need attention, student learning objectives, learning strategies and clinical practice evaluation criteria. It is signed by the PA and the student.

8. *English as a second language (ESL) teaching strategies*. This is included in response to clinicians' requests. Increasing numbers of ESL students participating in clinical cause concern. The session is about strategies for minimising confusion, understanding cultural nuances of different students, providing effective feedback to those students, understanding 'face-saving' issues, ensuring participation in the clinical area, emphasising that the onus for learning was on the students and highlighting adult learning principles for ESL students. This session is followed by an afternoon tea, allowing time for lively discussion among clinicians and academics about strategies to help ESL students with their communication skills.
9. *Feedback and assessment of competence*. The final session focuses on the critical issue of feedback and assessment of competence. This topic is fraught with hard questions and angst for clinicians, academics and students. The session focuses on assessment for competencies. It is particularly oriented towards more senior students effectively achieving their registration competencies. It is emphasised that in the second part of 2nd year and all of 3rd year, students are expected to meet the *ANMC Competencies* (ANMC n.d.) for their year level. At the end of 2nd year, students are expected to be using competencies for practice but only have a quarter of a workload. At the end of 3rd year, students are expected to meet the competencies in anticipation of registration and manage the full workload for a novice RN.
10. *Participant feedback*. At the end of the workshop, participants are asked for feedback to identify the workshop's strengths, where improvement is needed and suggestions for future workshops. Some examples of strengths identified from workshops are as follows: 'This really helped consolidate my knowledge and how to run the DEU'; 'Overall more understanding and appreciation of difficulties facing students—good session on supporting clinical learning'; 'Enjoyed ideas on giving feedback to students'; 'The Helpful Gatekeeper and feedback/assessment of competence'; 'The ease of interacting with the Lecturers'; 'Being able to discuss apprehensions of DEUs'; 'Great strategies to deal with specific problems' (Edgecombe 2010).
11. *Areas for improvement*. Examples of areas for improving the workshops include the following: 'More time on using competencies for feedback—important area'; 'Possibly have a student spokesperson'; 'Interaction with

students (present and past graduates) who can give us some suggestions about how to deal with problems in the wards'; 'I would like to see the laboratories and increase my knowledge of how the students learn there and the content of each course stage'; 'More role plays in how to provide feedback'. There was also a request to 'know where all the DEUs are and who are the PAs on my worksite, not just my area'; 'To maintain regular short courses/seminars for nurses who want to participate as a DEU in the future' (Edgecombe 2010).

Feedback resulted in advanced workshops for clinicians and PAs who were experienced in DEUs and later LN-specific workshops covering topics including how to deal with difficult students, clinical teaching strategies, providing constructive critical feedback and developing clinical learning contracts. Workshops were followed up periodically (fortnightly or several times per semester) with meetings/debriefings with clinical staff separate from the students.

Incidental Capacity Building for DEU Clinical and Academic Staff and Students

Reshaping the timing of clinical placements to privilege clinical equally with the theory of classroom work (Bail et al., Chap. 5, this volume) assists in incidental capacity building for all DEUs. The DEU structure sustains incidental as well as planned learning strategies. Incidental capacity building is a constantly evolving process that includes clinicians, clinical facilitators, students and patients in a collaborative learning process. For example, 'I have learned from the CLN and ward staff, and they have learned from me' (Elaine Horn, ALN, Manukau, Story 9, Chap. 10, this volume). The formal, planned structures (roles) in the DEU enable incidental learning in that they give a reason for maintaining a focus on the learning agenda. They generate increased research opportunities for academics and clinicians, opportunities for joint conference presentations and publications, and increased collaboration re curriculum and student assessment (Gonda, Chap. 4, this volume). The structures maintain guided feedback to students and academic guidance to clinicians for formative and summative assessment.

Clinical and Academic Staff: Support

Incidental capacity building can occur through informal staff meetings and PAs discussing with clinical staff topics such as current practice and research, student education, and standards and scope of practice (see Bail et al., Chap. 4, this volume). PAs may also discuss opportunities for learning strategies within the ward, such as visiting other departments or having clinicians run mini-tutorials. As discussed by Craig and Moscato (Chap. 6, this volume), at the University of Portland DEUs,

Clinical Instructors (CI) became more confident through their role as teachers and the support they received from academics undertaking the role of Clinical Faculty Coordinators (CFC); practice informed education and education influenced practice. CIs certified as expert clinicians gave scholarly presentations and assumed leadership roles on the unit. Some returned to school for a Master's degree or were promoted to leadership positions within their hospitals.

Students: Peer Teaching

Incidental student peer teaching across and within year groups, resulting from accommodating students across all 3 year levels in the same space at the same time, develops students' capacity as teachers and learners, guided by clinicians and clinical facilitators (academics). Thus, while the DEU is structured so that peer teaching is an intentional and supported strategy, peer teaching also happens to some extent by osmosis due to the students being together. The quality of the peer teaching is dependent on the quality of support. If the clinical staff and academics have the necessary knowledge and confidence to encourage and support students' peer teaching, it will become self-sustaining as students develop it more broadly: 'We were lucky because the CLN recognised the need for peer learning' (Taylor and Nand, Story 1, Chap. 10, this volume).

Conclusion

Clinical and academic staff capacity building is an integral part of the DEU design. As such, it is spoken about more as 'preparation' for or 'staff/faculty development' in the DEU. However, capacity building is greater than merely preparing clinical and academic staff, and students, for their roles within the DEU learning environment. It is about equipping them with professional skills that enable clinical staff to develop teaching as well as clinical expertise, enter academia or gain promotion within their organisations; academic staff to keep up to date with clinical knowledge and practice; and students to develop teaching as well as learning capabilities through peer teaching in DEUs. Clinical staff, academics and students develop the capacity to value each other's knowledge and to work collaboratively with an expanded diversity of peers and colleagues across academic and clinical settings/organisations. This type of capacity building underlines the possibility of interprofessional DEUs. Capacity building would extend across clinical and academic staff and students from different professions. Workshops expanded to include professions other than nursing could formalise the incidental cross-professional interaction that already happens in clinical settings. Student capacity building through peer teaching across different year levels achieves a variety of learning outcomes (formal and incidental). Therefore, a logical hypothesis would be that peer teaching in a DEU environment could accommodate the different learning objectives of different professions within that environment. Interprofessional collaboration is already implemented in one DEU in Sweden, where ambulance service personnel work alongside nursing personnel. However, research is needed into further interprofessional DEU possibilities.

References

ANMC. (n.d.). *ANMC competencies.* Australian Nursing and Midwifery Council. http://www.nursingmidwiferyboard.gov.au/Codes-Guidelines-Statements/Codes-Guidelines.aspx. Accessed 16 Aug 2012.

Benner, P. (1984). *From novice to expert, excellence and power in clinical nursing practice*. Menlo Park: Addison-Wesley.

Benner, P., Sutphen, M., Leonard, V., & Day, L. (2010). *Educating nurses: A call for radical transformation*. San Francisco: Jossey-Bass.

Bondy, K. (1983). Criterion-referenced definitions for rating scales in clinical evaluation. *Journal of Nursing Education, 22*(9), 376–382.

Cowan, D., Norman, I., & Coopamah, V. (2005). Competence in nursing practice: A controversial concept—a focused review of literature. *Nurse Education Today, 25*(5), 355–362.

Edgecombe, K. (2010) *Participant feedback*, DEU workshop. Adelaide: Flinders University.

FUSON. (1991). *Flinders University of South Australia (FUSA) submission for the Bachelor of Nursing Studies, Bachelor of Nursing (undergraduate) 1991—course proposals* (p. 20). Adelaide: FUSON.

McAllister, M. (1998). Competency standards: Clarifying the issues. *Contemporary Nurse, 7*(3), 131–137.

Chapter 10
Voices from the Coalface: The Impact of Dedicated Education Units in Nursing

Margaret Bowden, Anj Taylor, Vandhana Nand, Susan Randles Moscato, Jen Little-Reece, Thimitra Panteleon, Amanda Husslebee, Kylie Finlay, Paul Griffiths, Marina Boogaerts, Peter Mason, Tracey Duggan, Elaine Horn, Judith (Judy) Gonda, Ann Harrington, Kasia Bail, Sheona Watson, Cathy Andrew, and Mary Gordon

Glossary of Terms in Order of Appearance in This Chapter

Registered Nurse (RN) College- or University-qualified nurse licensed by a nursing registration body to undertake all facets of nursing in accordance with the body's regulations

M. Bowden (✉)
School of Nursing and Midwifery, Flinders University, GPO Box 2100, Adelaide, South Australia, Australia, 5001
e-mail: margaret.bowden@internode.on.net; margaret.bowden@flinders.edu.au

A. Taylor
Counties Manukau District Health Board, Middlemore Hospital, Otahuhu, New Zealand
e-mail: Anj.Taylor@middlemore.co.nz

V. Nand • E. Horn
Faculty of Nursing and Health Studies, Manukau Institute of Technology (MIT), Manukau City, New Zealand
e-mail: Elaine.Horn@manukau.ac.nz

S.R. Moscato
School of Nursing, University of Portland, Portland, OR, USA
e-mail: srmoscato@gmail.com

J. Little-Reece
Providence Portland Medical Center, Portland, OR, USA
e-mail: mjlittlereece@yahoo.com

T. Panteleon • A. Husslebee • K. Bail
University of Canberra, Canberra, ACT, Australia
e-mail: thimitra.panteleon@gmail.com; Thimitra.Panteleon@act.gov.au; amanda.husslebee@act.gov.au; Kasia.Bail@canberra.edu.au

K. Finlay • P. Griffiths
Ward 5E, Flinders Medical Centre (FMC), Adelaide, SA, Australia
e-mail: kylie.finlay@health.sa.gov.au; paul.griffiths@health.sa.gov.au

K. Edgecombe and M. Bowden (eds.), *Clinical Learning and Teaching Innovations in Nursing*, Innovation and Change in Professional Education 10,
DOI 10.1007/978-94-007-7232-8_10,

Clinical Liaison Nurse (CLN)/Dedicated Liaison Nurse (DLN)/Liaison Nurse (LN) an experienced Registered Nurse (RN) selected from the practice area who takes on extra responsibilities, including overseeing clinical learning in the DEU and liaising between staff, students and academics/faculty (particularly the ALN); the liaison between the unit and the University

Academic Liaison Nurse (ALN) a permanent clinical lecturer at the University who provides consistent support to students and clinicians

Principal Academic (PA) an academic lecturer in clinical (nursing school faculty member) who visits the clinical setting prior to student placement to facilitate clinical staff preparation for working with the students and thereafter visits the clinical setting regularly throughout each semester; communicates and liaises with students, the LN and the CNC, and utilises their ongoing expertise to facilitate students' learning

Clinical Nurse Consultant (CNC) in charge of the ward in which the DEU operates

M. Boogaerts
School of Health Sciences, University of Canberra, Canberra, ACT, Australia
e-mail: marina.boogaerts@act.gov.au

P. Mason
Division of Surgery, The Queen Elizabeth Hospital, Adelaide, SA, Australia
e-mail: peter.mason@health.sa.gov.au

T. Duggan
Canberra Hospital, Canberra, ACT, Australia
e-mail: tracey.duggan@act.gov.au

J. (Judy) Gonda
Faculty of Health Sciences, Australian Catholic University, Brisbane, QLD, Australia
e-mail: Judith.Gonda@acu.edu.au

A. Harrington
School of Nursing and Midwifery, Flinders University, Adelaide, SA, Australia
e-mail: ann.harrington@flinders.edu.au

S. Watson
Nursing and Health Studies, Manukau Institute of Technology (MIT), Manukau City, New Zealand
e-mail: Sheona.Watson@manukau.ac.nz

C. Andrew
School of Nursing, Christchurch Polytechnic Institute of Technology (CPIT), Christchurch, New Zealand
e-mail: cathy.andrew@cpit.ac.nz

M. Gordon
Princess Margaret Hospital, Canterbury District Health Board (CDHB), Christchurch, New Zealand
e-mail: Mary.Gordon@cdhb.health.nz

Clinical Coordinator academic responsible for negotiating clinical placements and ensuring placements are congruent with curriculum requirements
Charge Nurse nurse in charge of the clinical unit/ward

ECG Echocardiograph
BGL Blood glucose level

Clinical Service Coordinator the most senior nurse in the unit/ward; provides consultancy for clinical practice and management of all aspects of nursing within the unit

Clinical Nurse (CN) a Registered Nurse (RN) accorded a position of seniority and experience

Graduate Nurse Practitioner GNP

OSCEs Objective Structured Clinical Examinations to test students' practical clinical skills

Technical and Further Education TAFE

Enrolled Nurse Diploma qualified nurse working under supervision of a RN to provide nursing care

Charge Nurse Manager (CNM) takes responsibility for 'appointing' a RN to the Clinical Liaison Role (CLN) and rostering time for preparation, orientation and assessment as well as attendance at staff development/capacity building sessions

ANMC Competencies Australian Nursing and Midwifery Council competencies required for registration as a nurse (RN) or midwife (RM) (ANMC n.d.)

Non-government organisation NGO

Director of Nursing DON

Introduction

Dedicated Education Units (DEUs) in Nursing are essentially flexible student-centred clinical practice learning environments dedicated to producing more and better prepared nursing graduates whilst making optimal use of available resources. The diversity of definitions provided in the Introduction to this volume highlights different interpretations in different contexts. Despite the variety of definitions, all DEUs are based on similar principles: a fundamental respect for, and valuing of, human beings' individual and collective knowledge and experience; strong, respectful partnerships between universities and health-care services; a student-centred approach to learning; the development of key roles and responsibilities among academic and clinical staff within DEUs; thorough preparation of individuals undertaking those roles; ongoing teaching and clinical practice development for academic and clinical staff (capacity building); peer learning; and all participants in DEUs (students, clinical staff and academic staff) sharing knowledge. The principles enable DEUs to adopt different structures to meet the requirements of health-care organisations and University policies, organisational practice and ethos, staffing levels, funding levels, ward sizes, geographical location and the human beings who determine ward and health service cultures.

Continuing research into DEUs' performances is fundamental to their sustainability. The stories herein, which highlight issues affecting clinical education in DEUs and other clinical learning models, are presented in original form to maintain each contributor's voice. Some are written in the first person, others in the third person as observational pieces and others as conversations or interviews. The viewpoints expressed act as evaluations of diverse DEUs. Contributors have taken ownership of their roles within their DEUs, reflected on their experiences and expressed the desire to articulate what participation in their DEUs has meant for them. Story 5 in particular highlights the changing nature of a DEU over its 16-year lifespan and identifies issues arising over time that have impacted on how the DEU is run.

Stories are grouped in the following order by role to enable comparison of experiences across DEUs:

- Students
- New graduates
- LNs
- Clinical Nurse Consultants
- ALNs
- PAs
- Clinical Coordinators
- Executive

Student stories are presented first to reflect the DEUs' student-centred approach to learning. There is no analysis of individual stories. Interpretation is open to you.

Students

Story 1: Our Voices Were Heard

Anj Taylor and Vandhana Nand, 3rd year DEU students, Manukau Institute of Technology (MIT), New Zealand

Anj and Vandhana have come to nursing as a profession after working in very different non-nursing environments. Anj had been an executive chef, working in a fast-paced, people-driven, communication-oriented environment in London. Vandhana had been working in a diagnostic lab, isolated from much communication with other people. Both were so inspired by the DEU concept that they applied, with a sense of privilege, to be part of the Manukau DEU in New Zealand. Here they share their DEU experiences.

If there was one thing that we really hated being referred to in the clinical setting, it was 'the student', for instance 'Do you want the student today?' or 'Get the student to do it'.

In the DEU we were not called 'the student'; we were welcomed as valued members of the nursing team.

We've changed a lot already through the feedback sessions, and these changes have been put in place for the next DEU. We feel so valued; 'our voices were heard'.

Anj: When I was first introduced to the concept of the DEU, I felt inspired by its philosophy, and I was excited to not only have a chance to experience a new way of learning but also be part of MIT's DEU Pilot programme.

Vandhana: The lecturer introduced the DEU concept in class and I was interested because it was such a new concept, so I put my name forward. I was surprised not many students took the opportunity to take part in the DEU. The idea of having the lecturer alongside you in the ward was a factor that pushed me to take up the DEU placement—this offered quality teaching and support.

Anj: In the DEU everything was transparent from the start. We had a thorough orientation, so everyone knew what to expect and what was expected of them. *We knew where we were going, we got to meet all the key people in the ward, were shown the ward layout*. The orientation helped us to be more familiar with the ward environment and helped to make us feel more at ease on our first day.

We had a sense of belongingness. We were embraced straight away as part of the team. We weren't considered outsiders. We didn't have to prove ourselves. From day one we were involved 'within our scope of practice'. There was no opportunity for failure because there were people there to help you all the time. I didn't feel lost or lonely or disheartened like I had in other placements.

In my previous placement, students were seen as the 'booby prize'—not wanted. Nurses made this so obvious. But in the DEU, students were really wanted.

Nurses were even 'bagsing' students—because they wanted a particular student. It got to the point where some nurses were moaning they didn't have students. We were valued as an additional resource.

Another thing that made me feel really part of the team was that I broke my arm halfway through placement, so I couldn't come in and do anything, but I was called in for teaching sessions and tutor sessions so I was still learning. As soon as the cast came off, I finished the hours in the holiday break. The nurses were so happy to have me back. They were saying, 'It's so good to have a student'.

Vandhana: The ALN and CLN need to be proactive—and they were. They helped students with their learning. They were both very well informed. They had excellent knowledge. Also, our ALN treated everyone at the same level—*there was no favouritism*, which can happen sometimes. Whatever learning she gave to one she gave to another. On a personal level, if a student asked for help, that student would get help. Students were encouraged to ask for help, and even though students were responsible for their own learning, the CLN did a lot of work for us—she went out of her way to get other people to run small sessions with us.

Another good thing about the ALN and CLN being right there was that you could talk to them if you had any problems.

I had one bad experience in my first week in the DEU. I was with a nurse who was brilliant at what she was doing but I couldn't keep up with her. I was not ready for this. So I told the CLN the problem. The next week I was put with someone else and it was much better. It was great to have someone there on the spot to talk to about issues and who *listened to what we were telling them.*

Anj: The ALN was a valued member of the team. Although she was a tutor, she was also a RN and she was embraced as part of the clinical team very quickly as soon as she came into the ward.

The ALN and CLN were in the clinical setting all the time, which meant they were able to set up learning experiences; because of this we felt that we were really advantaged, so we often refrained from talking about our experiences to other students, because we felt that they may feel disadvantaged because they weren't getting the same opportunities.

The clinical tutor was there all the time, on the spot, and would take students aside and help them learn—it was very positive teaching.

Assessments were accurate because the ALN was there all the time and could see everything.

Vandhana: *I think the assessments were harder because the tutors were there all the time. With other students, assessment was just a process. It was not going on all the time.*

Anj: In a normal placement, assessment happens at the midway point, and then action plans are created to adjust the students' learning if necessary. There's no need for this in the DEU because *adjustments are being done all the time*.

Also, there is peer learning.

We were lucky because the CLN recognised the need for peer learning.

There were three different years in the same environment. The peer learning was invaluable. No one was afraid of feeling dumb. For example, 3rd year students may help the 1st year students to understand a concept that they might be struggling with. It was good to have a group because it's so easy to get lost when you are the only student rattling around in a big ward, like happens in some placements.

Vandhana: As students, we were so comfortable with each other; if anyone had any problems, they were happy to ask another student for help, or other students would offer help. *It was like a family.* There was no competition between the students to be higher than each other—everyone was willing to help.

Anj : The ALN recognised the need for students to have space for their own learning—students would often take over meeting rooms for independent discussion. The ALN made students stand up and be real nurses. She wanted the students to know everything about a patient, which led to involuntary teaching moments with the patients because the students had researched everything about them. We were in a ward where terminal diagnoses were common, and researching the patients' condition gave us an awareness of the patients' situation.

The ALN gave us just the right amount of support. Sometimes we needed emotional support and the ALN was right there when we needed her.

Vandhana: The support we had meant we were not overwhelmed. We didn't feel, 'Oh, what are we doing here?'

Anj: During our placement, we had a nurse who had a needlestick injury who wouldn't report it because she was scared she'd get into trouble. We had a group of three students discussing the ethics of this and decided it had to be reported for her own well-being. So we did.

We had so much SUPPORT.

The ALN understood what we were learning, what our expected outcomes were. She had the competence to take us to a teaching moment. She would gather up all the students and take us, so we didn't miss the moment. And she worked with the CLN to give students as many learning experiences as possible.

You were supported and pointed in the right direction. *You felt like a real RN.* By the end I was looking after four patients. On an individual level I needed a four-patient load to keep me stimulated. If I had downtime, I talked to patients and got too attached. But the CLN and ALN recognised students' individual levels and we worked according to that. No one in the ward frowned upon anyone who could only manage a two-patient load—*it was all individual levels.* The RNs appreciated the students taking over patient loads because it freed up some of their time to give better care to a lesser number of patients.

We had learning objectives; a lot was centred on getting to know patients and doing assessments. The patients loved it. They got a lot out of the students when the nurses were rushed. Sometimes all the patients needed was someone to listen to them. And they would ask for you by name. It made us feel really valued.

Vandhana: When I started nursing I was worried, 'How will I communicate with people?' *In my first placement, for two weeks, I was on my own and I found it difficult to connect with patients. In my second placement, which was in the DEU, I had no trouble connecting with patients.* I had a lot of Maori patients. And all I was worried about was cultural safety, cultural safety, cultural safety! But *I had support all the time,* and I learnt that patients are all basically the same. If you say, 'Hi, how are you, etc.', they are happy and they say that to you too.

I had a patient who was part of a gang and when I talked to him, he seemed like a nice man. Then he told me about him killing people but I didn't feel scared. I had a good nurse-patient engagement with him.

Anj: You feel comfortable in your environment.

Everyone wins in the DEU. The Charge Nurse was excited because she was picking students she wanted back as RNs. And the students got great learning.

Story 2: It Changed My Life!

Susan Randles Moscato, then Associate Dean and Professor, School of Nursing, University of Portland, Oregon, and Jen Little-Reece, DEU student at the University of Portland, Oregon

Susan and Jen recount an experience they shared at a DEU conference held in Portland, Oregon, in July 2008.

In the usual clinical, the clinical day consisted primarily of me observing the nurse do various procedures . . . and [the nurse] didn't even remember my name!

In the DEU, there was no downtime, no observational time; just practice time.

Susan: This story comes from Jen Little-Reece. Participating as a panel presenter for the conference, Jen decided that her unique contribution would be to talk about what it is like to be a student on a DEU and contrast that with her experience on a unit that was functioning in the traditional clinical education model and assigning students to a different nurse each day.

Jen began with a description of what she experienced after six weeks in a 'usual' clinical.

Jen: Typically, the Charge Nurse took the students around the unit and introduced me to my nurse for the day. The nurse had already been in report and was checking lab values at the computer. She told me to follow her, took me into the first patient's room, introduced herself, then *introduced me as "a student nurse working with me today"* and proceeded to do an assessment. After she was finished, she invited me to listen to the patient's lungs whilst she worked with the IV and managed various pieces of equipment. The clinical day consisted primarily of me *observing the nurse do various procedures, and scrambling, digging and scratching to get the clinical experiences I wanted!* The nurse didn't know what I was able to do or how safe I was in doing any particular procedure. *She didn't even remember my name.*

Susan: Jen then contrasted her experience in the traditional teaching model with practice as a student nurse on a DEU.

Jen: I got to the unit for report, after which my Clinical Instructor (CI) asked, 'What's your plan for the day?' I shared my plan and headed out to the computer to check labs. *When I walked into the first patient's room, I introduced myself as the person who would be providing care, then introduced my CI as the person who would provide me with support as needed. I was in charge*, did all of the work that was needed with assistance from my CI and spent my time fully engaged with delivering care. There was no downtime, no observational time; *just practice time.*

Susan: Jen summed up her experiences by saying that having the same nurse for six weeks allowed her to be *'completely and utterly supported'* by her CI, who knew her strengths and knew when to push so that Jen would learn more.

Jen: My education on the DEU allowed for an *in-depth evaluation of my abilities* that would be impossible on a traditional unit. The life changing education I received on the DEU wouldn't be possible without the close relationship I developed with my CI. The DEU is clearly perfect in every way! *My education on a DEU was crafted for me*, to make me excellent.

Susan: Jen brought tears to the eyes of people in the audience when she said, *'It changed my life'*.

New Graduate RNs

Story 3: Ready for the Transition: Returning to the DEU as a New Graduate RN

Thimitra Panteleon, newly graduated Dedicated Education Unit RN, Canberra University

Thimitra reflects on the advantages of Dedicated Education Units for better preparing students for their role as professional nurses.

We had already been given a chance to familiarise ourselves with how the ward works and its rituals.
The DEU prepares you accurately for what to expect once you are on your own.
The transition itself feels as though there is not so much pressure to impress or prove yourself.

Throughout the DEU final placement, confidence is gained through understanding the ward routine, the staff members who are to become colleagues, the workload, shift work, the role of RN, your own boundaries and the satisfaction of working as an RN.

Understanding the ward routine is a big component because within each ward there is a different environment, and we had already been given a chance to familiarise ourselves with how the ward works and its rituals.

As students, we work with different RNs and get a feeling of what kind of nurse we want to be. Having already worked with staff members who are to become colleagues, you have already worked out who your mentors are. Through this, when working as a new grad, you are able to focus questions and ideas towards the RNs whose responses you have confidence in as accurate and professional.

In regard to workload issues, the DEU prepares you accurately for what to expect once you are on your own. This was also true for preparation for shift work. Although it was hard to get used to, throughout the DEU experience you are given a fair taste of late-early shifts and how to cope and prepare for them. It was all part of preparation for the transition from student to RN.

The transition from student to the role of RN feels as though there is not so much pressure to impress or prove yourself. The rest of the team have got to know you quite well in the prior six months whilst you were learning in the DEU, and they know your capabilities and areas that need improvement. I really feel like this is a major advantage over the other new grads who started their new grad placement in an unfamiliar area.

Knowing your own boundaries is very much attained throughout the DEU, and it gives you a chance to speak up when feeling out of scope as a new grad. I don't feel as though I would have been able to say 'no' if I didn't understand my expectations from other wards.

Finally, the DEU gave me a sense of comfort in my surroundings, which added to my level of satisfaction of working as an RN. If I was not so comfortable in my surroundings, I am sure a plethora of doubt would have made the experience as an RN not so enjoyable.

I am very grateful for the year in total I spent on 6A. I was prepared and ready to start my new grad experience, and that was entirely because of the way they made me feel as a final placement student throughout the DEU.

Story 4: Grounded in the DEU: First Days Back on the Ward as a New Graduate RN

Amanda Husslebee, newly graduated DEU RN, Canberra University

Amanda talks about how her Dedicated Education Unit preparation for becoming a graduate RN helped her concentrate on 'being a nurse'.

I started to fully comprehend the responsibility inherent in the role of a RN.
It really struck me how fortunate I was to have been on the ward before now.
I could explore what this new role meant for me both personally and professionally.

I remember feeling relieved when I found out who my preceptor for my first day was. I knew from working on the ward as a student that she would be kind to me and let me work at a pace that was comfortable for me. After a while, I was able to stop focusing solely on how to get through the shift and more on how to get through the shift with good time management, doing everything that needed to be done competently and safely. This was made easier by the fact that I had been on the ward as a student so I had a basic understanding of the ward routine. It was just finding my own routine that took some time and refining. It was at this point that I started to fully comprehend the responsibility that is inherent in the role of an RN. The fact that I was out practising on my own with no one to watch over me or answer to was an intimidating and overwhelming realisation. This was when it really struck me how fortunate I was to have been on the ward before now. It meant that I knew far more than I credited myself for: things like where to locate everyday objects that you need to function throughout a shift, for example, Obs/ECG/BGL machines, treatment room, code to the locker/handover room, staff toilet, public toilets and phone numbers; also, how to respond to common 'problems' seen on the ward, such as low BGLs, high BGLs, 'chest pain'; and when, and who, to call for help. I really felt that already knowing these little things allowed me to concentrate on 'being a nurse' and what is expected of you in that role (and how that differs from your role as a student nurse). It also meant that I could explore what this new role meant for me both personally and professionally.

Liaison Nurses

Story 5: Let's Trial It: The First DEU

Kylie Finlay and Paul Griffith Flinders, Medical Centre (FMC) DEU, South Australia

Kylie Finlay and Paul Griffith were members of the original DEU pilot at Flinders Medical Centre (FMC), South Australia. Kylie graduated from Flinders University in 1993 and completed the Graduate Nurse Programme at FMC in 1994. She has worked on the GI Unit (Ward 5E) for 16 years and has been the unit's Clinical Service Coordinator since 2005. Paul Griffith, who had been an RN for approximately 19 years when the first trial DEU began in 1997 in Ward 5E, was the first DEU Liaison Nurse (LN).

They talk about their experiences from the time of the first DEU in 1997 in Ward 5E to the current DEU in the same ward.

We trialled the DEU and it's still here.

I think the DEU allows students to feel part of the team, whereas with a block, the students are sort of just here and gone.

I see them every week over the 16 weeks or six months. So I get to know them ... and they get to see their families each week, whereas with a six-week block, that takes up all their time and all our time.

Having experience with both block and DEU, I prefer the DEU for the knowledge aspect—understanding WHY, not just rote doing things, not just knowing how.

Some of the nurses on the ward were DEU students when I was the LN... they're back now and they've been working on the ward for years; we're reaping the benefits.

I've also done the PA role, which was very beneficial.

We have a duty of care to our patients to make sure our nurses are safe.

We can get them to understand the academic side, but getting them to do the practice is completely different.

We've now got less time to teach. In the old days we had a lot of time for teaching, especially with staff members who have English as a second language.

I don't think either block or DEU placements prepare students for shift work.

Kylie and Paul: Peter (Mason) made sure there was a teaching culture in our ward; we had good RNs who were good nurse teachers, who were enthusiastic about teaching students coming through, and we went along with what Peter said, so we trialled the DEU and it's still here.

Kylie: It's something Peter was involved with, and so being RNs on his ward, we trialled it with him.

Paul: Well, because we were the first ward to trial it, one of the issues we had at the time were students doing morning, afternoon and night shifts, so at times students were without a liaison person. I was the first Liaison Nurse (LN). Even though we had people to support students, if there were problems, we'd sort them out the next morning when I was back in, so to start with, there was not always an LN available on all shifts. That was in the old days—you just took what you got and got on with it. Now we have one dedicated nurse who works Monday to Friday for the semester. And there's only the morning shift and the late shift.

Kylie: This makes it easier for continuity but it's harder from a ward perspective because you're taking that nurse off night duty, so from a management perspective, it is more difficult. I think it's really good to rotate—we have always rotated the LN role. We originally did it for a year, but we went through a stage where we just didn't have anyone really senior enough to take on that role. People had already done it, so we got to the point where people had got a little bit burnt out. People didn't really want to do the LN role again, and there wasn't really anyone suitable for it. That was then. Now, we're back to the stage where we've got lots of people who are trying to develop their Clinical Nurse (CN) staff portfolios, so it's a very good situation.

Paul: It would even be good to put junior staff members there because they'd still have the support of 20–30 other staff who have already done the LN role; but not be totally new, because it is very stressful to the RN that's doing it every semester.

Kylie: It's been really good. Some of the nurses on the ward were DEU students when I was the LN, so that's where Julie[1] gets all her skills—from me! Yes, so they're back now and they've been working on the ward for years.

Paul: They're nurses that I've actually taught myself and they're now the more senior nurses and they are fantastic nurses. No issues of concern at all.

Kylie: What Paul could have said was actually that 'I taught you, then you taught what I taught you to Julie', but that's OK.

[1]Not the name of a specific student; a random name chosen to represent many students not referred to individually.

Paul: We are reaping the benefits.

Kylie: Absolutely. I think if they have a good DEU experience, and everyone has put into the students, then they actually request to come back to the ward during their graduate year and then they request to become permanent staff members through their experience. We've got a couple like that. And I think coming here to do the DEU settles students into their graduate year because they're accountable for a full patient load whilst they're doing their placement, and a lot of them come back. It's not such a shock, as this is a busy surgical ward. They've actually been here and they've spent six months here.

Paul: But then sometimes they do experience that culture shock, because before when they were students, they had somebody to fall back on: a supervisor. Now they have to settle in reasonably fast, especially on this ward, and look after personal patients. They still have to be supervised but not in such a role, and they are a bit more stressed at times. But then, we are all busy working and it's mainly checking things.

Kylie: We've all been liaisons, had our turn. I remember I felt burnt out when I did the DEU LN role because I was also doing the acute med-surge course at the same time and I think I had a six-month-old baby. So that's why I was burnt out—not related to that role. It was all the other factors.

Paul: I didn't get burnt out. My philosophy is if I can train a good student to become a good RN, then I've done my job. That's what it's all about—training good students to become good registered nurses to look after patients now, and my parents and myself one day. I've also done the Principal Academic (PA) role, which was very beneficial as well. It was very rewarding because we also got nurses out of the DEU for that to count towards Graduate Nurse Practitioner (GNP). And also, I think I pushed a bit more because we have a very high standard on this ward and I thought I didn't want to be the PA who failed any nurses. Well, I did fail one. We put in a lot of work and even though we wrote in specific times, he just didn't come back, so...

I didn't have any training to be the PA. Basically, Judy Gonda approached me and said, 'Paul, I'd like you to do the PA for the next semester, next six months'. No problems there. 'This is what we expect, here's your paper work, you've got these liaison people at the University'. *We had a great time doing that as well.* My basic contact was with Judy. There was more nervousness on my part because I didn't want any student to fail. I did the PA role in the last semester so the students had to do their viva or OSCEs. I really drilled them for their OSCEs.

The University contact people changed whilst I was PA, and they had very different ways of doing things. One was relaxed in her approach but was very tough and very strict. You knew who was going to fail and if you didn't know your stuff, you'd get a bit of a kick and you went out there and pushed the students really hard. 'You listen to the staff because that's where you're going to get all of your hands on and all your experience'. I got used to working with the first contact person. Then the new person took over the role. She had a very different style, much more academic, whereas the first one was more hands-on clinical. After about the first or second semester, the new person came round to the way we did things on our ward and she was fantastic. I think she was a fantastic academic as well. It was a bit of a culture shock between the two of them. Different personalities, different styles, but we worked well together after the settling in period.

Kylie: Definitely different styles. One was more hands-on clinical whereas the other was more theoretical, academic, and now we've got another one, and she's lovely; she just fits in, does what she has to, communicates . . .

Paul: She will come up and say, 'Paul, Fred is failing in this area, we need to get him to work with a certain number of staff members there', which we try to do; but that's the fine line because they're at the end of the semester here and there's not a lot you can cover in time.

Kylie: The communication about students has changed a lot over the past 20 years. We went from not talking about students . . . like a talking about students behind closed doors sort of approach where we'd just go through and discuss each student and their progress, and now we have an approach where we . . . we haven't done one for a while, have we Paul?

Paul: No. I feel out of the loop at the moment; there doesn't seem to be much communication.

Kylie: I just thought of that. Well how are they finding out what the students are like?

Paul: After we had the communications in the seminar rooms behind closed doors, we went to a writing formation, so at the end of the shift, we'd write something about the student we were working with and give that to the liaison person, who would then tell the PA. Then we went from that to the students giving us their appraisal forms at seven o'clock in the morning to plan for the afternoon, and then it was verbal, and now . . . The only real communication you get from the University is if you fail a student.

Kylie: Yeah, *we must talk to the University contacts* and find out how they are getting accurate feedback.

Paul: Yeah, because the only time I know something is if the University contact person comes and tells me about particular students who need extra help.

Kylie: You expect students to have different levels of knowledge; 2nd year, I think, it's about information, knowledge, gaining hands-on knowledge. Third year's about time management and understanding why they're doing things; they should already have the knowledge.

Paul: Responsibility.

Kylie: And really getting them prepared to be walking out, as a first day graduate, knowing that they've got four patients and planning for them.

Paul: I had a 2nd year the other day who was standing by the nurses' station saying they had nothing to do. So we took her and gave her some patients to do hands-on stuff, and she wasn't hanging round the nurses' station again...

Kylie: Over the years, we've had to drop back on the numbers of DEU students we've been getting each semester because we're busier than ever. Often when the DEU students aren't here, we're being asked to fit in a three-week block placement, which is often December, which I'm now saying 'No' to because we're just burning out with the constant demand the health-care system's putting on all of us. If it's not block placements we're managing refresher RNs, re-entry RNs, overseas nurses and also TAFE ENs. We're managing a lot. We've dropped from 12 DEU 3rd years down to 8 DEU 3rd years. Three years ago I had to write to the University because we were so efficiently run we were being allocated a lot of overseas DEU students and that was really difficult. We've also had to cut back on the number of overseas nurses as well. It was just their comprehension—about them saying 'Yes, yes, yes' to everything but not understanding what we're saying.

Paul: I suppose in all this, too, this ward has really changed. We don't get any light acuity patients any more. It's all high acuity now.

Kylie: Major abdominal surgery we're doing now.

Paul: So we've now got less time to teach. In the old days, we had a lot of time for teaching. And especially now with staff members who have English as a second language, it's frustrating. You think, 'We've been here already; do we have to explain it again?' It's so time consuming.

Paul: Right now the issue is with the students. They get allocated the patients, which is not an ideal formula in regard to understanding what wound they're looking after—knowing the diagnosis, knowing the medications, knowing the patients, how to communicate, how to settle into the ward, and then making sure that when the PA comes around, they're able to give her adequate feedback and information without having to spend a lot of time on the computer. We have allocated 30 min time-out every day to read up, to get up, to speed with everything about their patients, but that 30 min can extend to an hour if they're not supervised. But then you've got to appreciate too that they are supernumerary and they are learning.

Kylie: I feel the staff need to have a break from students—just to be able to come on and look after your own four patients without having to check everything. It's nice occasionally not to have a student load.

Paul: Yeah, definitely.

Kylie: I don't think either block or DEU placements prepare students for shift work. You know, sometimes they do it, but the late-earlies, and the night duty and the weekend work, which is what they don't have as students. You know nursing is a very shift work-oriented profession, so they don't actually get the feel for it, what it's really going to be like, going home and having four hours sleep because it takes you three hours to unwind. They don't get the real experience.

Paul: Some want to do nights but we've said 'No'.

Kylie: We need a rest too.

Paul: But when you come to December, and you're finished with the DEU students, you've got quite a few who have had days off, to get their paper work done, their essays, so they extend a little bit further and a little bit further so we don't end until two weeks later. And then we'll get hit with a block...

Kylie: Yeah, which isn't good. We're quite burnt out.

Paul: I don't think the DEU is more time consuming than the block.

Kylie: The issue is having both. No one wants to take on a block and a DEU; no one wants to put their hand up to do that.

Paul: In the old days, we used to have the Mondays, Tuesdays, Wednesdays, with Thursdays and Fridays off, but then we lost too many days through public holidays on the Mondays, so we swapped it over. We found that Monday also was student-free—we could relax, you got all your work done on time; you didn't have to explain. *We're not getting any extra money but what you get in benefits out of it is that you care for teaching*. It's an issue of timing, too, of when students are in the ward.

I find the DEU run over the 14–16-week period is the ideal, except at the beginning because you're here for two days then you're away for five, then you're back again for two, and all the things you've learnt in the first week, you've forgotten by the second week. But then they start to remember by the third week, and they start to get a foundation base to build on, and then they start to build on top of that, so by the time they leave between the 14th and 16th weeks, we've got a pretty good idea of whether the student's going to be a good RN.

With a block, I find because it's such a concise and restricted period in the six weeks, you give them so much and I think they find it very hard to accept all of that. I suppose a lot depends on the nurse then, whether they're going to be a good nurse or whether they're just going to be mediocre. Also, the students are here all the time so we don't get a break. It's nice to get a break. There's so much to do in such a short concentrated time.

Kylie: I think nursing's a lot about common sense. If you haven't got common sense, then you're not going to be a good nurse. I think the DEU allows students to feel part of the team, whereas with a block the students are sort of just here and gone, and it's just a job, which probably led to a bad experience recently where what comes back from the students doesn't fit with the amount of work put in. We had a very good LN, and we put a lot of work into the students, and not even one of them gave us a card of acknowledgement when they left. Normally some of them do. This is the cultural thing that comes in where students just expect it's your job, whereas a lot of work went into that first six months with some difficult students, and now it's sort of as if that's all it is.

Paul: That's not the first time that's happened. When one of the other LNs did their six months, to be told by students, they hadn't taught properly and there was no support; that was unfair. There's definitely a difference between a first semester student and a second semester student.

Kylie: Yes, I just think over time . . . it's more like they're doing us a favour more than we're doing them a favour. I think it's generation Y. They work to live, not live to work like some of us.

Paul: Yeah, they do. There's not a lot of thanks at the end of the day, except for occasionally from us guys. I think a lot of it stems from whoever's the Clinical Nurse Consultant (CNC) on the ward and what their ward culture is. I think this ward's got a great culture; great learning ward, great teaching. Our standards are very high and that sets us up very well.

Kylie: I think we do set very high standards and we expect that from students on the ward. If that were me in the bed who was sick or one of my family members, I'd expect high standards.

Paul: And it's making sure that you understand the patient's signs and symptoms, and knowing what you have to do and when to do it.

Kylie: You have to keep them alive. It's about being able to identify when patients are unwell and acting accordingly.

Paul: If you've got good teachers, then the students are generally going to follow suit, except for some overseas students who go, 'Hey, I've seen this before', but it's come from seeing an unqualified person in a different country, and they try the same thing here where it doesn't fit with our culture. And when you ask them where they're going to go to work, if it's back to their teaching hospitals over there, they're not going to do things the way we teach them. It's a different culture.

Kylie: Which is difficult again because we put a lot of work into these students. They come over on visas.

Paul: Absolutely. But I have the greatest admiration for the students who have English as a second language because they try so hard. They convert language to language, and then they try to talk to the patients and you're there to support them and the patient. They try so hard but you've still got some of those old guys that just hate Germans and Japanese regardless because of the war history, saying, 'Get out of my country'. There's their cultural way of learning too: they've got the books, they've read the literature, they've got some understanding, then you've got to try and teach them the Australian cultural way, at the bedside, hands-on, and then you've got to make them understand at a standard you think is acceptable and safe. And then you've got to make sure the patients are OK with it, and the student has to know what they're doing, and at the end of the day, they can put it in context, be critical of the literature, can write it all up and then be quizzed by the PA and can say, 'Yes, this is what I had to do, and this is how I found all the literature about it, and this is how I put it into practice in a hands-on context'. We can get them to understand the academic side, but getting them to do the practice is completely different.

I think that one thing with learning and teaching and patient care that I'm always trying to improve on is how I can communicate. Not just me. I listen to the other staff in the ward and how they communicate with each other, and to the patients, and then to the students—how they get that information over to the students and what the student understands and what the patient understands. I listen to how all these people chit-chat. Sometimes it doesn't work, so I pull everyone back and say, 'Maybe I was explaining the situation this way', which makes it a little bit easier, but sometimes we don't have that luxury. And sometimes you get three different people showing students to do something three different ways; maybe three generations of people.

Kylie: One of the domains now in the clinical nurse portfolios is to demonstrate clinical teaching. So it's good to have that down as a portfolio item. It would be good for the universities to actually acknowledge a DEU LN. I get them to keep the dates and it would be good to have a certificate to say they've done this. You know, because the portfolio is such a big thing these days. It would have to go at least towards your clinical nurse reclassification.

I think you've got to be wary when you are a DEU that you don't focus all your time on your students and forget about your grads, especially if you've got a few difficult students. That's happened before, where the grads have been left. Paul's our graduate liaison here and it was difficult when he was trying to do both because it's too much to concentrate on.

Paul: I have a split focus. In the block, the graduates are just here for six weeks, here and gone; I might not even see them. If they are a better standard at the end than at the beginning, then I'm happy. At the end of six weeks they've done what they need to do and so have we. I feel like six weeks is not long enough to get a good GNP, but they have to be a better standard at the end of it than when they come.

In the DEUs, I see them every week over the 16 weeks or six months. So I get to know them—different personalities, where they've come from, and they get to see their families each week—whereas with a six-week block, that takes up all their time and all our time.

Kylie: With the DEU, you're likely to work with the students, but with the block placement, if you've been on annual leave, you might miss a whole batch of students.

Paul: With the DEU, if there is a problem or a concern, you've got a longer time to work that out. But with the block, again, because it's at the end of the year, clearly the next year they're supposed to be RNs but it doesn't give you a lot of time to get a nurse out.

Kylie: When I completed my block placement as a student, I came out of it with no knowledge at all; it was just basic nursing care. I honestly believe I had no knowledge, and luckily I'm a fairly common sense person and that's what's got me through. And you know you develop knowledge as you go, obviously, but I really don't think I took any knowledge away from my block placement. It was like, 'I'm here, I know how to do a bed wash and that'. But I think the DEU allows students to progress to understanding what they're doing, not just doing it; to understand nursing.

Paul: The DEU progresses from one to two to three to four bases, whereas with block, you haven't got much time to orientate them and get them to the coalface before they go. In a DEU, you can tell whether students are going to make it or not. If not, you speak to the PA and put the student on a contract; then, if they fail, they fail.

Kylie: Our younger LNs really worry; they want everyone to pass, but we have a duty of care to our patients to make sure our nurses are safe. If students in their graduate year show signs that they won't be a good nurse (when they can't do the simple common sense things) then it's our duty to make sure this is addressed. In the DEUs, 3rd years must be able to practise at a safe level. We will not sign off on students we feel are not safe. Any problems, we talk with the PA, LN, staff members and students. We don't get many problems on this ward. We don't go making mountains out of molehills. We've got so many senior staff members on this ward who have done the DEU that we have a very high standard.

Paul: I had one bad experience once where what a student did was potentially dangerous. I yelled 'Stop, stop, stop!' 'Whoa, what did you just do wrong?' I explained what they did right and they knew what they did wrong. They didn't do it again. We have a duty of care to our patients to make sure our nurses are safe to practice; and a duty of care to our students.

With the DEU we don't have too many horror stories because we can see the situations before students fail and there's time to work on issues before they become problems.

Kylie: Yeah and you know they're going to make it and if they're not, you get the PA involved and you either put them on a performance plan or they just go and never come back because obviously nursing's not for them. It doesn't matter how good a teacher you are, some people aren't going to be good nurses.

Paul: A lot of our liaisons, especially our young liaisons, worry and stress. And I say, 'Guys, why do you stress? You've got the best ward, nearly everybody's done DEU liaison, there's so much help there, you've got the PA coming across there... In regard to whether you've got six or 26 or 36 students, it's a very simple procedure'. They want to make sure everybody passes.

Kylie: And we've got a duty of care too in our profession to make sure that nurses that are unsafe don't get through because we've also been on the rebound of having some very average graduates, that we've had to... one I think we had to go to the Nurses Board for, one we had to go to senior management for because they've just not got it when they've graduated and you think, 'How did this person get through?' And I think we really need to be honest to our profession.

Paul: Yes, and how are they going to affect our standard? We do have a high standard here.

Kylie: Yes, but the ones I'm talking about here were simple, common sense things that you just think, 'How did they get here?' And you know, after that 3rd year student placement, you do pick up problems. You don't let them go until they're registered and then say, 'Oh, hang on . . . '.

Paul: You can't teach common sense. But it's getting harder and harder to fail people. We're watching the safety aspects, with our patients especially, and they thank you at the end of the day. We don't get many issues on this ward and I think that's because we can follow through from first year. I'm not saying it's the be all and end all, but it works pretty well.

Kylie: Having experience with both block and DEU, I prefer the DEU for the knowledge aspect—understanding WHY, not just rote doing things; not just knowing how.

Story 6: A DEU in 'Invisible Nursing': From Hesitation to Strong Partnerships

Marina Boogaerts, Adjunct Professional Associate Community Health with the School of Health Sciences at the University of Canberra, Australia

Marina is a DEU Liaison Nurse (DLN) in Australian Capital Territory (ACT) Health Community Health DEU. She is also a Clinical Nurse Consultant (CNC) at ACT Health Community Health Continuing Care Program. She reflects on the development of partnerships, relationships and student and staff learning in Dedicated Education Unit learning environments.

There was a sense of working together.
Seeing students turn the initial 'chat' into 'assessment' was very satisfying.

I have worked as the DEU Liaison Nurse (DLN) and been involved in the Community Health DEU since the model was introduced in the Australian Capital Territory (ACT). Whilst initially the model met with some hesitation from certain areas of community health, it evolved into a strong and valued partnership.

Students in the Community Health DEU participated in community-based nursing services such as maternal and child health clinics, school immunisations, alcohol and drug services, prison nursing and generalist community nursing. The students had the unique opportunity to experience nursing in a nursing-led environment, which was underpinned by a philosophy of primary health care, harm minimisation and wellness. Nursing in these areas is often 'invisible'. At the start of their placement, students often had difficulty defining the nursing work. They would use phrases such as 'the nurse was having a chat with the client'. It would not be until a few weeks into their placement that the layers of the nursing work would become clear. Giving students the time to take their experience away, reflect and discuss with peers and academics, and then come back week after week, developed the richness of nursing in the community. Seeing students turn the initial 'chat' into 'assessment', 'using the right questions to get the information needed' and 'looking for opportunities to empower the client' was very satisfying in my role as DLN. This was only possible because good relationships existed between the Principal Academic (PA), the students and the clinicians.

A DEU Reference Group with senior representatives from the clinical areas, students, the PA and the DLN met regularly to discuss goals and experiences. There was a sense of working together. This was particularly useful in the community setting because clinicians and students were spread out across the territory. It also gave the group an opportunity to articulate the positive effects the model had on staff. Attendance at the meetings was high and a number of collaborative projects resulted from this group.

Clinical Nurse Consultants

Story 7: Win, Win, Win

Peter Mason, 'the clinician who is passionate about the DEU'

Peter is currently Safety, Quality and Risk Management Coordinator, Division of Surgery, The Queen Elizabeth Hospital, Adelaide, South Australia. He reflects on his time as the Clinical Nurse Consultant (CNC) in the first DEU at Flinders Medical Centre, South Australia.

The theoretical model is only as good as the people implementing it—it's all about the people.

It was having people who were passionate about the DEU way of providing clinical education that made it work.

I don't think I'll be able to teach anyone else because I don't know anything.

It was the best! She just knows such a lot.

It was a win, win, win situation: a win for the academics, a win for the students and a win for the clinical staff.

I was the Clinical Nurse Consultant (CNC) in a very busy gastrointestinal surgical and medical ward (5E) at Flinders Medical Centre when Kay Edgecombe and Judy Gonda from the Flinders University School of Nursing approached me to ask if our ward would be part of a pilot for the Dedicated Education Unit (DEU) model of clinical practice teaching and learning. I have always been passionate about finding better ways of doing things, so I felt privileged to be asked to be part of a new way of developing students as nurses. I was excited by the DEU and, as CNC, was proactive in getting it approved by the organisation. Having trained in the hospital system, I felt that the DEU could combine the best of that system with others—it could provide a longer time for students to model themselves on staff and learn how a health-care team functions.

Previously we had had the traditional block placements, which were not ideal. All the staff in our ward shared a good focus on student education and were vocal about what was working and what wasn't. The general consensus was that block placements did not give students the experience of staying on a ward for any length of time and they did not experience how a health team really functions. Nor did they feel part of that team. Staff felt they did not have adequate input into the students and there was no sense of continuity in watching the students develop. We wanted students to see the broader picture over time rather than a snapshot of what makes health care effective.

I got all the staff together and we talked as a group about the possibility of running a DEU. We saw that the DEU could give the ward clinicians greater input into role modelling for coaching the students. Some staff had reservations. They were afraid the DEU would make their life harder. They feared the sheer volume of people that would be on the ward. Like everyone, they asked, 'What's in it for me?' I think initially there were a lot of non-believers. But all staff were given the opportunity to input into the pilot.

We decided to go ahead. I talked to management and explained the DEU philosophy and how this new way of doing things could work in the gastrointestinal surgical ward. They said 'OK'.

All the staff recognised that when the students first came into the ward, there would be a lot of extra work and a lot of extra people. Initially, the staff felt overwhelmed. The nurses had an increased workload and the nurses' station was like a train station! But we knew if we put in the effort to start with, we would reap the rewards later; and we did. We really wanted the students to develop a sense of working as a team. When I orientated the students, I said, 'We want you to be part of our team'. Some looked a bit confused. I don't think they'd had this invitation before. I really think it was important for them to feel a sense of belonging. But they also needed to understand what this meant. So we spelled this out to them. For example, one of the things that annoyed the clinicians was students sitting at the nurses' station and not answering the phone ringing or not doing anything about a patient's bell ringing. Students seemed to think they weren't allowed to take any action because they didn't know everything. We explained to them that they didn't need to know everything but they could help by answering the phone and saying, 'I'll just go and get someone to talk to you', or attending to the patient bell. By working as a team, we successfully changed both the nurses' and students' attitudes; both came to realise that students could help. Similarly, we overcame the problem of an overcrowded nurses' station by asking students to go to another room to read case notes.

Previously, the academic facilitator would breeze in and breeze out, saying, 'I'm just going to see the students. Where are they?' With the DEU, there was a much more focused approach where we utilised an experienced clinician from the ward—

a Liaison Nurse (LN) who acted as a clinical learning facilitator/coach/mother hen 'go to person' for students, academics and myself as CNC. The LN was always available. This role was integral to the success of the DEU process.

A lot of the staff struggled to come to terms with the idea of peer teaching and learning. As we moved through the DEU process, peer teaching and support, in which 3rd years teamed up with 2nd years, and 2nd years teamed up with 1st years, created unease. Most staff held the belief that the more senior you were, the better teacher you were. However, after thinking about this and seeing the students in action, we realised that we had been expecting graduate nurses to teach and support students, but the graduate nurses had no previous experience of doing this. We came to see the benefits of helping the students develop these skills from the beginning.

I'll always remember one 2nd year student who had minimal clinical experience. This student worried a lot and was totally overwhelmed by the complexities of the ward and the thought of teaching other students. She came to me and said, 'I don't think I'll be able to teach anyone else because I don't know anything'. This student was paired with a 1st year student who gave a completely different picture of the 2nd year student's abilities when I asked about their peer learning experience. The1st year student said, 'It was the best! She just knows such a lot'.

Students gained a greater understanding of what was required to be a nurse, which enabled us to step back later and let the students practice. We constantly discussed the issue of how much leeway to give the students. But if you look over their shoulder all the time, they don't develop. You can't expect them to make the quantum leap from 3rd year nursing student to graduate nurse if they haven't had the chance to act autonomously or semi-autonomously. Our aim was to get the students working at graduate nurse level before they left the DEU; they would do medications and handle a full patient caseload. For example, students were asked to come and check medications with the RN at an appropriate time. If they missed that time, they'd be given a prompt. Having the students manage a full patient caseload freed up nurses' time to do other things. We turned the tables a bit. For example, nurses always wanted to go to theatre but there had never been time for them to leave the ward. Students, when they first came to the ward also wanted to go and see surgery. So, we would send them once, and then, when they had progressed to taking a full patient caseload on the ward, we could send the nurses. The nurses felt this was an enormous benefit and a reward for all the hard work they had put into the students initially.

I developed a very strong relationship with Judy Gonda and Kay Edgecombe from the Flinders University School of Nursing through the DEU. They used to roll me out as 'the clinician who is passionate about the DEU'. There was barely a month when they didn't bring someone visiting from overseas to talk with the staff, which really made the staff feel important. The relationships between the clinical and academic staff are so important. The theoretical model is only as good as the people implementing it. It was having people who were passionate about the DEU way of providing clinical education that made it work. When we implemented the DEU, we had a larger number of students on the ward than other wards because we were willing to take them—up to 18 students a day over two shifts. Working out ways of managing these extra people in an already hectic and crowded environment required flexibility and constant problem solving. But having a dedicated team of people helped. If there were any problems, we sat down and talked about them. It was not just left to me as CNC to come up with a solution. Staff came up with ideas and we worked out what would work best.

Staff and students were given the opportunity to provide feedback about the pilot DEU as they progressed through it, which heightened the sense of teamwork and belonging. The LN was a critical person in this process. Staff and students felt comfortable going to the LN if they had any issues, because this person was part of the ward and part of the team.

The most important experience for me was the ability to combine the best of what the clinicians could offer with a strong academic process. Exposure to these two together made the students' experience much stronger. We had a passionate DEU PA and the majority of the nurses were passionate about it too because they were asked for their input. The DEU helped me develop a clearer understanding of the students and gave me the opportunity to identify future staff; students who could come back and work with me once they were qualified. The number of students who benefited is obvious by the number I employed back on the ward. It was rare for us to have outstanding vacancies because DEU students, once they graduated, were keen to fill these. I think the DEU provided them with a unique experience in which they recognised staff were committed to educating them.

I think the DEU contributed to improved outcomes for the students. I definitely think it is a superior model to the block placements. But I have had conversations with people elsewhere who don't like the DEU. It comes back to the people and the context. It was right for me and it was right for our ward. Feedback from the staff and students also indicated it was right for them. The staff were very proud of being the pilot DEU. They saw it, and so did I, as *a win, win, win* situation; a win for the academics, a win for the students and a win for the clinical staff.

Story 8: Tears and Fears, Joy and Pride: We Miss the Students When They're Gone!

Tracey Duggan, Clinical Nurse Consultant (CNC) of an Acute Medical Ward Dedicated Education Unit (DEU), working in collaboration with the University of Canberra

Tracey recounts the value of having students in the clinical setting over an extended period of time.

So many students on the ward at once can be challenging.

Students become part of our nursing radar.

We know their strengths and what supports they need: they are not another 'unknown'.

We see students as part of our workplace. We miss them when they're gone! Not only do we enjoy meeting them, sharing our passion for nursing with them and watching them grow and learn; we also rely on their help with our work, as well as how they keep us on our toes! I firmly believe in the shared learning that takes place within a DEU. However, having so many students on the ward at once can be challenging, particularly space-wise. But by having them with us every day, we are always aware of them and their progress; they become part of our nursing radar, so it is easy to communicate with the University representatives about how they are going. We are sad to say goodbye to the students when they have been with us for six months; it's a bit like children leaving home. You've shared tears and fears, and joys and pride with them; you learn so much together. Some of our students come back as new graduates and that is great, especially when you have put in the hard work to support them. It also works well because we know their strengths and what supports they need: they are not another 'unknown'. And they are more confident coming back to us. They have less stress because they know the skills mixes, the personalities, the patient types, the medications, common clinical pictures, the doctors, social workers, etc. The DEU offers great satisfaction for my work—to see students transition, both personally and professionally, into nurses.

Academic Liaison Nurse

Story 9: The Clinical Reinvention of Batman and Robin

Elaine Horn, Academic Liaison Nurse (ALN), Manukau Institute of Technology, New Zealand

Elaine reflects on how her trepidation at taking on the ALN role turned into a fulfilling experience.

Life [in a DEU] becomes so much easier.

I have come to love the sense of belonging.

I have learned from the CLN and ward staff, and they have learned from me.

Through my feelings of belonging and comfort in this ward, I am better able to work as a team member to enable student learning.

My life as a nursing lecturer used to be lonely, with no real sense of being either a member of the nursing team or one of the students. For the last eighteen months, it has been very different.

I began working as an Academic Liaison Nurse (ALN) on a busy medical ward in a large public hospital in Auckland, New Zealand. There were 12 students from each year of the three-year Bachelor of Nursing programme—more students in one ward than I had ever had to cover. *How was I ever going to cope* with assessing their competency, facilitating their learning and ensuring that they see nursing as the amazing profession it is?

Part of this 'experiment' is the role of the Clinical Liaison Nurse (CLN). *She turned out to be Robin to my Batman.* How? Well, the CLN and I work together to ensure that the students' learning needs are being met, that they feel supported and that they are progressing. We regularly discuss students' performance with each other, with the Charge Nurse Manager (CNM) and the registered nurses who have the students working with them. Life becomes so much easier. *No wandering around looking for nurses with little time or inclination to discuss students with you.* I spend my entire day and working week on this ward. I now know all the nurses by name and level of experience, the other members of the interdisciplinary care team and the medical team. This NEVER used to happen when I visited the five or six wards I had students scattered around in previously.

Initially, I thought I would hate being in one ward because I used to enjoy the flexibility and mobility that comes with covering several wards. I have come to love the sense of belonging and I am certain that through this I have become better able to assess student performance and facilitate valuable learning experiences. *I have learned from the CLN and ward staff, and they have learned from me*. That has to be a win-win situation. My nursing and clinical assessment skills have been utilised in the ward, which helps to build my credibility as an experienced Registered Nurse (RN) and educator. *Through my feelings of belonging and comfort in this ward, I am better able to work as a team member to enable student learning*. A student once described that she 'felt like one of the family' in this placement—so do I.

Principal Academics

Story 10: We Are All Learning from Each Other

Judy Gonda, Principal Academic (PA) for the first Dedicated Education Unit (DEU) developed by Flinders University, South Australia

Judy is currently an Undergraduate Course Coordinator, International Advisor and Senior Lecturer, School of Nursing and Midwifery, Australian Catholic University, Queensland. She reflects on her PA role in the early days of DEUs.

After only the first semester in the DEU I started to feel like part of the team—I always knew what was happening at the coalface.

We didn't always see eye-to-eye.

A small community where everyone (students, clinicians and academics) is continually learning from each other.

I was the Principal Academic (PA) for the first DEU developed by Flinders University in collaboration with Flinders Medical Centre in Adelaide, South Australia. I was there for seven years and two things stand out for me from my time there. The first is the relationship I developed with the Nurse Unit Manager,

Peter Mason, and his nursing team. The second is the cultural change that occurred over that time. These were quite different from any of my previous experiences.

I have been actively involved in clinical education for 15 of the 21 years I have been involved in nursing education. During those years, I was involved with the 1:8 clinical teacher to student model, the cluster approach and finally the DEU model. In the 1:8 and cluster models, I always felt like a visitor in the wards, and one who was mostly endured resentfully.

After only the first semester in the DEU, I started to feel like part of the team. I was welcomed when I arrived on the ward, invited to morning tea and lunch with the ward staff and included in all the usual ward gossip. Consequently, I always knew what was happening at the coalface—the issues surrounding staffing levels, skill mix, changing practices and how all these were impacting on the nurses in the unit. In short, I felt like I belonged and that I was accepted as a nurse rather than being viewed suspiciously as an academic. The students observed this on a regular basis and I believe it gave them a positive perspective of the relationship that can exist between academics and clinicians.

Peter and I had a similar philosophy about what was important for competent and caring nursing practice, which made it easy to work together right from the start. In addition, we were both absolutely committed to making this DEU into the best learning environment we could. This had a positive trickle-down effect on the rest of the team.

However, Peter and I didn't always see eye-to-eye. The thing is, we always seemed to be able to come to some consensus about issues where we diverged. I believe this was because we had a relationship based on mutual valuing and respect. I valued him for his knowledge about current nursing practice, and managing a complex team of nurses and patients as well as the hospital organisation; and he valued me for my educational knowledge and my understanding of the curriculum and the University organisation.

A particular issue that comes to mind was how we decided to set up the Liaison Nurse (LN) position in our unit. I wanted the person to be in the position for at least two consecutive semesters so that there would be some consistency and the incumbent would have time to develop into the role. I was viewing it primarily from the individual's perspective and how that person would liaise with me as the PA. Peter wanted a different individual in the position every semester because he saw it as an opportunity to prepare his staff members for leadership roles and a privilege to be offered as a reward for those who demonstrated potential. He also felt that if a number of the staff had been in the position, they could support each other in the role.

We decided to go with his idea initially, with some doubt on my part, and see how it worked. If it didn't work, we'd go with my idea. It turned out that his knowledge of what motivated his staff was correct. We changed the LN every semester. In no time at all there was a critical mass of nurses in the team who could support whoever was in that position. In addition, we never had a problem filling the position. It seemed to be viewed as something to aim for by aspiring Registered Nurses (RN).

Over the seven years I was on the unit, I saw many changes in the ward culture as a result of having the DEU, but one aspect was particularly rewarding. Right from the beginning, we had staff meetings every two weeks to talk about any problems arising from the implementation of the DEU and to discuss individual student progress. Any nursing staff member who could take time away from patient care was encouraged to come and we always had a good turn up.

Initially, I would find these meetings a little disheartening because the comments about students were often very subjective and judgemental—'she's fantastic' or 'he's hopeless' were common statements—but they were often said with no objective substance. I would try and ask them for some evidence of why they were making these statements to try to determine whether the judgements were based on personality clashes or whether they related to actual competence.

I started to introduce the *ANCI Competencies* as a way of giving the staff a framework for evaluating the students objectively. They were familiar with these competencies for student assessment but, like most clinicians, saw them as a tool applied by universities rather than hospitals, and therefore they had not systematically applied them with any conviction of their usefulness.

Over time, I saw that it was not me who was asking, 'Which competencies do you think this student has a deficit in?' It was the nurses on the unit. In addition, it gave them some scaffolding to help students who needed it, for example, they'd say, 'If they have a deficit here, we can do this, this and this to help them overcome it'. Essentially, over time this changed the focus of the meetings and the unit culture to one of nurturing the students rather than passing or failing them. Consequently, we had many students placed on Clinical Learning Contracts on the unit, but most students passed because the staff used the contracts to help the students learn and improve rather than to fail them.

This has to have been one of the most pleasurable experiences I have had in clinical education, and to me it epitomises what the DEU concept is all about; a small community where everyone (students, clinicians and academics) is continually learning from each other.

Story 11: From Bad to Brilliant

Ann Harrington, Clinical Researcher, School of Nursing and Midwifery, Flinders University, South Australia

Ann talks about her experiences in setting up one DEU and taking on the PA role in another.

I had the time to really get to know this student.
The situation went from bad to brilliant!
In the DEU, I learnt from the clinical staff and they learnt from me.
It was all about trusting and letting go.

I have always been passionate about clinical practice and was involved in Dedicated Education Units (DEUs) for six years. The DEU has more going for it than any other model. I have been involved in block clinical teaching, hospital teaching and cluster clinical teaching as well as DEUs, but for me, the DEU provides the most supportive environment for the students, as well as academic and clinical staff in developing future nurses. In my opinion, it is far superior. Students become totally involved; they are nurtured and become part of the team. Even if students come with a negative attitude, the DEU provides the time and space for the Principal Academic (PA), Liaison Nurse (LN) and other clinical staff to work with them in a controlled, supportive environment that can turn negative attitudes into positive progress. Students get to know other students and the staff and can translate a lot of what makes them nurses into the clinical setting. The DEU makes the links between University work and clinical practice; this is why the PA is so important. The PA provides the students with the guidance to achieve this link.

I set up my first DEU in the operating room at a community hospital in Adelaide. My role was to liaise with the DEU Coordinator and the perioperative staff in day-only wards, general surgical wards, the recovery room and general theatres. The hospital staff and I wrote perioperative standards for students, aligned with the *ANMC Competencies* (ANMC n.d.), so students knew what they had to do. It gave them a template of objectives for their period of placement. This provided an evaluation tool for students and staff. The evaluations came back incredibly positive.

Whilst still involved with this DEU, I took on the role of PA in a DEU in a palliative care setting. Palliative care is unlike the 'biomedical model' in its approach to care because the person/people in the patient's family situation is the centre of care. Consequently, the care that students give often taps into their own humanity. I did two days per week in each location. After several years I handed over the operating room DEU to someone else and continued two days per week in palliative care (I did the 'front' and 'back' of the DEU).

My experience in the perioperative DEU and the palliative care DEU has reinforced the unique care philosophies of these two very different areas of nursing. The perioperative care 'follow-through' philosophy involves following the patient through from the pre- to the in- to the post-operative stages. Students in the perioperative DEU would introduce themselves to the patients before they went for their operation and would reassure the patients they would be there with them all the way through. The patients loved it.

The same follow-through process would happen in the palliative care DEU when patients had to go to theatre to have a PEG feed inserted. But within a hospice there is the added relationship building of patients returning home and then returning to the hospice, so students got to know them really well. And dealing with death had a major impact on some students. It unlocked unresolved grief from earlier personal experiences. I worked with these students, as did all the staff, to help them work through their feelings. If needed, I arranged counselling for them. This really helped them in their clinical practice. It was the kind of attention that's not possible in a block placement.

I had one student who felt the whole world was against them. They were very negative and had a history of making it difficult for anyone to work with them. When this student came to the DEU, I thought, 'Oh no. Here's the potential for a very bad situation'. I wasn't mistaken. In the first few weeks, they complained that the DEU wasn't taking their special learning needs on board, they couldn't learn anything in palliative care, it was a waste of their time, they should be doing proper nursing…

The good thing about the DEU is that *because the person from the University is there every week, they can address this kind of problem before it gets too big.* I organised a meeting between myself, the LN and the student to talk about the philosophy of palliative care and the student's issues. I made sure I was on the unit at handover time so I could talk to this student, who needed a lot of attention. I had the time to let them vent, as I knew they needed to do this. The benefit of the DEU was that *I had the time to really get to know this student* and work with them to overcome some of the issues that had impacted on their progress. There was also *time to build solid relationships with the staff* and get them on board in helping the student. At the end of the DEU, this student, who had initially decried clinical in palliative care as 'useless', came to me and told me how much they 'loved palliative care!'

So, *this situation went from bad to brilliant.* The student even came back to do Honours. They had been able to tap into things they were good at and had responded positively, over time, to the nurturing setting of the DEU because I, and the staff, had taken the time to work with them.

The therapeutic setting of the palliative care DEU and the time provided to work with the students every week helped me develop the students *personally* as human beings and *professionally* as nurses. It was important that students were working with good mentors, and that they were on the DEU long enough to develop as part of a team, and to make connections with patients and staff over a long time. Students had to write objectives every day based around the *ANMC Competencies* (ANMC n.d.) to prepare them for aligning themselves with the Competencies and professional registration. This approach was not always popular. One student said it was 'a trial' but I said, 'It is your foundation for practice', so the student did it.

I couldn't be there all the time so I had to trust others to provide a University education in clinical. I liaised with the staff regularly to make sure they were aware of the Competencies and that clinical practice is about competence, not tasks. The students were not just to be allocated tasks and shown how to do things. As well as showing students how to put a catheter in, for example, clinical staff were to explain why the patient needed a catheter, what else was going on for the patient in terms of things such as how they would cope psychologically with the catheter and what's going to happen if they go home with the catheter in.

In the DEU, *I learnt from the clinical staff and they learnt from me.* In the palliative care DEU, we'd have in-service seminars. The staff were wonderful. *The RN would listen to me about professional issues and I'd listen to her re clinical practice.* I learnt to trust the clinical staff. *It was all about trusting and letting go.*

Addendum

I am now reaping the rewards of the long-standing, respectful relationships I developed in the palliative care DEU in terms of current research in palliative care and oncology. I am publishing with a clinical nurse with whom I worked in this DEU. We continue to skill-share in linking grants and collaborative research projects between the palliative care organisation and the Flinders University School of Nursing and Midwifery. I currently have one collaborative project running there and have had two others over the years. I am working with the staff to produce more as I see no benefit of research if this doesn't translate into practice. My attitude as a clinical researcher is: 'Nothing should stop the development of research'.

If I were asked to go back to do DEUs now, I couldn't as the pressure of research is too great. The reality is I am now a nurse researcher and although I have contact with clinical staff, I no longer have involvement with the students.

Story 12: 'Walking the Talk': Reflections on the Principal Academic Role in a Dedicated Education Unit

Kasia Bail, nursing lecturer, University of Canberra

Kasia reflects on the PA role in one of the Canberra DEUs, highlighting how this role helped her develop as a clinical lecturer.

Being a Principal Academic made my new role as a lecturer make sense.

It was always opportunistic, discussing issues that were right in front of us.

I found it so fascinating that I was constantly drawn to discuss things I noticed with other academics.

The DEU enables moderation.

As a newly employed academic, I struggled with the role of 'lecturer'. I enjoyed teaching nursing students, I enjoyed sharing my enthusiasm and delving into topics, I enjoyed learning about constructive alignment in designing curriculum and assessments. But, I struggled with the 'sage on the stage' environmental structure, and I found it difficult to bring my detailed memories of patients and their stories into the unfamiliar lecture halls and tutorial rooms. I often felt like I was fighting with students to help them understand the brevity of their role in making patients safe, to help them see the relevance of assignments and homework to patients' lives.

However, being a Principal Academic (PA) made my new role make sense. On a weekly basis, I was embedded once again in the messy clinical environment; I could work side-by-side with the students and walk them through what they were working within—either unpacking what they noticed about clinical practice (exploring their questions) or helping them to notice different aspects of practice (getting them to ask questions). Sometimes this was with one student, sometimes a group of students of different levels, sometimes it was with clinicians or both students and clinicians. Sometimes it was about disease management, sometimes hospital management, sometimes patient trajectories or multidisciplinary communication. It was always opportunistic, discussing issues that were right in front of us. And then I found these weekly engagements could feed back into my classroom teaching in the form of both storytelling (helping students learn from other students' experiences) and curriculum design. Working with students and staff in the field made it apparent to me what our curriculum lacked, where it was strong and which student patterns of study created different outcomes. I found it so fascinating that I was constantly drawn to discuss things I noticed with other academics, thus creating a community of practice within our hallway. The DEU enables authentic constructive alignment both at a unit level (for each subject the students studied, which included clinical assessment) and across the degree (as the assessment included the *ANMC Competencies* (ANMC n.d.) so the students could see how they were progressing towards registration).

The DEU enables moderation; students are assessed with input from the PA as well as the clinical team. Additionally, the hallway discussions offered another opportunity for moderation. The DEU enables formative assessment. The PA involvement in designing structure and expectations means there is support for formal and informal feedback, one of the biggest areas of complaint in student clinical experiences. The DEU enabled me to actively participate in collaboration with clinical areas; not just rhetoric, but active, weekly engagement. It allowed me to offer my expertise in research or higher education for the clinicians, separate from supporting them to support the students. The DEU fosters a shared approach—that nursing students are our future and our shared responsibility.

The weekly face-to-face contact and collaborative work towards integrating theory and practice makes me feel I am 'walking the talk'; that my role in the DEU gives authenticity and relevance to my role as a nursing academic.

Clinical Coordinator

Story 13: Putting the 'Action' into Action Research: The Counties Manukau District Health Board (CMDHB) and Manukau Institute of Technology (MIT) 'Action Group'

At the time of writing, Sheona Watson was a Lecturer/Clinical Coordinator, Nursing and Health Studies, Manukau Institute of Technology, New Zealand

Sheona recounts her experience as a key player in evaluating the establishment of two inpatient DEUs that were partnerships between the Counties Manukau District Health Board (CMDHB) and Manukau Institute of Technology (MIT).

There was a real sense of partnership and collaboration between members.

We didn't win a prize but were very pleased with our efforts.

The Counties Manukau District Health Board (CMDHB) and Manukau Institute of Technology (MIT) 'Action Group' was set up in 2009. The name was chosen as it seemed to fit nicely with the year-long action research project that was being used to evaluate the establishment of our two Inpatient Dedicated Education Units (DEUs). The members of this group—the Charge Nurse Managers (CNM), the Academic and Clinical Liaison Nurses (ALN and CLN), along with the Undergraduate Coordinator from CMDHB and the Clinical Coordinator MIT—were key players in the project because the DEU, by nature, requires close cooperation and communication between the educational and clinical providers. *We thought 'The Action Group' was a very appropriate name* as we felt that we would be generating much of the data that would be evaluated.

We held weekly one-hour meetings. The purpose of our meetings was to:

- Co-ordinate day-to-day operational issues within the DEU areas
- Monitor student/staff satisfaction
- Facilitate staff communication regarding the processes in place
- Provide feedback and support
- Participate in action research

The first meeting allowed the group to get to know each other and start planning for the clinical orientation day, which is such a key aspect of the DEU. There was much work to be done throughout the semester and the group members were totally committed right from the start. There was a real sense of partnership and collaboration between members, and *individuals were happy to contribute, knowing that all ideas and suggestions were considered equally.*

The collegial nature of the meetings allowed for debate and discussion of many issues, both clinical and academic, that are impacting on nursing practice within the DEUs. This was hugely worthwhile but often meant that some items needed to be followed up by email as we hadn't quite got around to them in our discussions. The learning we all took away from these meetings was very beneficial to us in our individual roles. The interaction also allowed for *frank discussion of student progress and local processes or factors that may impede student learning. The varying viewpoints allowed us to come up with innovative solutions.*

We also *managed to find time to socialise together*, partly to celebrate our successes but also to continue to grow as a group. Just as students were telling us they felt a real part of the nursing team with a keen sense of belonging, the same was true for the members of the Action Group. We were keen to spread the word about the project and the DEU concept, and prepared a poster submission for the local Health Board 'Sciencefest'. This called for a few extra meetings but the group was determined to showcase our work. With the *pooling of our individual talents*, the poster was designed and submitted, meaning another evening out as a group at the event. We didn't win a prize but were very pleased with our efforts.

The ALN and CLN from the community DEU were able to start attending the Action Group meetings. The group has already proved to be a useful forum for all to discuss issues from practice and now will have the benefit of a slightly different take on possible solutions to issues raised. *The geographical distances that the ALN and CLN have to travel must have implications for them getting together, but we hoped the action meetings would give them another opportunity to catch up to discuss any student/practice issues.*

As ever, meetings started with much discussion re current issues in practice and day-to-day concerns of the hospital/community. It is often like this. We worry that we will not get all details attended to, but this open discussion and collaboration is what the DEU concept is all about and a natural progression of the workings of this group.

Another unique feature of the DEU was *the opportunity for peer learning and support. This was a hugely satisfying aspect of the project* and the topic of much discussion at the Action Group meetings. With students of different levels in clinical at the same time, peer learning was optimised. Every student had an interest in each other's learning and the DEU philosophy allowed them to check on each other's progress.

The *positive support from the CNMs* during the pilot has had a huge impact on the project's success. Their individual contribution to the group has been invaluable. Each has embraced the ideas, found ways to work around any issues that have arisen and interacted as excellent role models with the students. The *growth in the CLNs* has also been an exciting factor in the project. The role is definitely a step up for senior RNs on the floor but with the support of the ALNs and our regular meetings, they have made exciting progress, moving from individuals who were unsure how to move ahead to confident clinical leaders.

Our regular meetings have been influential in the success of the pilot and we would strongly urge anyone establishing a DEU to consider a similar set-up to oversee the project. It was pleasing to know that they wanted the Action Group to continue at the end of the pilot without a name change! The team members felt they were indeed the ones providing the action and that it was an appropriate name to use going forward. As much as it is *the role not the person*, the gelling of personalities has certainly made this action group a very worthwhile aspect of our DEU model.

How is the DEU experience different from that in other clinical learning placements? Here, students, lecturers and clinical staff share their experiences of working, teaching and learning in different DEU environments.

We now (2013) have 12 DEUs and are assisting Waikato DHB and Wintec in their pilot DEU project so we are all keeping busy.

Executive

Story 14: Out of the Silos into Inter-organisational Partnerships: Leadership, Vision and Collaboration

Cathy Andrew, Head of the School of Nursing at Christchurch Polytechnic Institute of Technology (CPIT) and Mary Gordon, Executive Director of Nursing at Canterbury District Health Board (CDHB)

Cathy and Mary talk about their roles in forming the CPIT/CDHB DEU partnership to address concerns about the quality of clinical learning for undergraduate nursing students.

When people first hear of the DEU, they think of it as a physical entity, rather than a set of principles.

The 'status quo' was not an option.

The DEU has the potential for wider application than nursing.

It wasn't about either organisation but about solutions that would benefit nurses and impact positively on patient care.

The DEU can adapt to meet the practice setting needs.

I am struggling to think of any disadvantages of the DEU model.

There has been a change of attitude towards student nurses by the practice environment.

As a student nurse, Cathy had had personal positive experiences as a comprehensive student. As a Registered Nurse (RN), she had noted that students were not often integrated into the team, for example, little things like writing names on the board and allocating times for morning tea. This observation stimulated ongoing thinking about how students could have better experiences whilst on placements: 'I always carried that with me throughout my nursing career . . . how could we work together so that students have a better experience?'

Mary had recently returned to Canterbury and had noticed some very constructive relationships at individual levels between some clinical practice settings and some education lecturers, but there was not a comprehensive relationship throughout either organisation (Canterbury District Health Board or Christchurch Polytechnic Institute of Technology—CDHB or CPIT). There were silos working very effectively, whilst in other areas there were limited relationships. The 'status quo' was not an option to continue for Mary, and, 'As a nursing leader I couldn't stand by and let the then situation of *them and us* continue to impact on not only the nursing profession but also the health system of New Zealand'. Mary became aware that a number of senior nurses, including nursing leaders; nurses employed in designated senior positions such as Charge Nurses, Nurse Educators and Clinical Nurse Specialists; and experienced and expert RNs, believed that the students exiting Bachelor of Nursing programmes were 'not for purpose'. Students were seen as a burden and not safe to be on busy acute hospital wards because their presence added to RNs' stress and distracted them from patient care. Others believed it was not safe for students because they would not be able to cope with the busy acute clinical environment.

Mary and Cathy both noted an increasing trend of Charge Nurse Managers (CNM) cancelling clinical placements at late notice (some even as short as a few days before students were due to commence their clinical placements). CPIT (the local education provider) were attracting students but increasingly not having enough clinical placements for them to complete the minimum required practice hours. This situation also translated into very few new graduate nurses being employed within the CDHB. However, a pilot had just commenced for new graduate nurses called the 'Nurse Entry to Practice' programme, which offered a supportive programme to transition the newly qualified RNs from being a student to being a competent RN within 12 months.

Cathy originally found the Flinders University research and talked to Mary about the DEU concept for about 18 months before moving forward. They asked themselves, 'How do we create positive learning experiences for student nurses?' They looked at various learning models. They were aware that something needed to be done. It was clear that, like other health professional workforces, nursing was going to face shortages with the increased population demands and the fact that Canterbury's population was likely to face this impact before other parts of New Zealand. Mary stated, 'If we did do not take every advantage to attract students into nursing, then we would not even replace the current workforce. Professionally, I believe that I have a responsibility, as does every RN, to ensure our next generation is well educated and trained, and the undergraduate preparation and transition to practice years are the basic infrastructure required to build and develop a highly effective nursing workforce to meet the changing health needs and service delivery models that will evolve to meet the population needs. It is this infrastructure level that is vitally important to invest in so that post registration and postgraduate education and development can be well leveraged to extend, expand and develop advanced nursing practice'.

Cathy and Mary made a commitment to work in partnership to change the way their organisations worked together. They had a joint goal of improving the nursing students' experience on clinical placement and of addressing the issues reported by both the students and the staff working in the clinical practice settings.

However, they had to wait for the right people to come along and for them to have the potential (to incorporate it) in their roles. A staff member from the School of Nursing (CPIT) with a passion for student learning in practice approached Cathy, saying, 'I need a project'. In order to be successful, representatives from both organisations were needed to explore a range of options together. A working group (WG) was established, consisting of two nurse educators from practice (District Health Board—DHB staff) and two nursing lecturers from education (CPIT) to look at the concerns and how these could be addressed. Mary observed, 'The working group were all committed to teaching and also to practice, which I believe was one of the key successes. Thus, it wasn't about either organisation but about solutions that would benefit nurses and impact positively on patient care'.

Another key factor that shaped the DEU evolution was that the WG was given an open brief; there were no predetermined solutions. However, there was recognition that this was not a problem unique to Canterbury. Therefore, others must have attempted to solve these issues. The WG had a disciplined approach to addressing the project brief and were forward thinking. They could see the potential for a wider application than nursing, for example, their principal statement as part of the logo was ‘supporting clinical learning’. This meant it could be applied to interprofessional learning within a practice setting. In addition, the WG were given the authority to utilise action research methodologies throughout the pilot and evaluation so that outcomes were underpinned by an evidence base.

Mary and Cathy, as leaders of their respective organisations, provided support, guidance and commitment, as well as strategic leadership, for the setting up and implementation of the DEU model in Canterbury. Cathy stated, ‘I wanted the DEU model to work as I had a sense it was going to mean that students had positive clinical experiences’. Cathy had to be creative in resourcing nursing staff time to work on the DEU model because no additional resourcing was available. At the same time, workload equity had to be maintained among staff in the school to ensure the school as a whole was committed to the model.

Mary spoke about being an ‘enabler’, providing governance oversight and being a permission ‘giver’. She was also in the unique position of being able to influence the local nursing leaders to support the model, not just within the DHB organisation but within the Canterbury Health System. Mary also had to gain organisational support not only from the nursing profession but more importantly from the wider health system. This included support from board and executive management level of the DHB all the way down to the clinical practice settings and across the organisation and health system, such as support from the finance teams, clinical board, middle/service management and partnering organisations such as the community nursing providers/NGOs.

The practicalities of introducing and maintaining the DEU model cannot be underestimated. ‘When you have a new idea, it is hard to understand how it will work and it is so important to get it right’, Cathy said. The DEU has been shaped and evolved into an identifiable package by the commitment of all involved.

Key aspects identified for a DEU included:

- Strong leadership within both organisations committed to the DEU to gain support from senior nursing staff and senior management staff
- A Working group with a mandate to work on the implementation and maintenance of DEUs and an annual work plan as to what they need to achieve
- A Governance group where policy decisions and any barriers or issues can be resolved
- Opportunities for working group members to present at conferences and be involved in research that maintains stimulus for the model
- Dedicated time for the CLN to prepare for and orientate students and undertake student assessments
- Regular workshops for new DEUs and new CLNs/ALNs

- Celebrating DEU success, such as coverage within the organisation's media and communications plan
- Successful DEU and student experiences increasing demand for areas to become a DEU

As we have progressed through the exercise of developing and implementing the DEU, some of the challenges have been staffing. Staff turnover is common in any organisation. We have had positive stories of the benefits of consistent staff and it appears that it is an advantage to the student. Cathy commented, 'Students have articulated that the assessment process is fair and valid. That is a major achievement in an environment where the professional judgements of RNs around the clinical competence of individual students are increasingly placed under scrutiny through appeal processes and challenges. Another advantage is that we have been able to respond to requests by the DHB to increase the number of students accepted into the programme. We have been able to do this with a level of confidence that the quality of clinical learning will not be compromised for students on placement, even though the numbers have increased significantly. At a professional level, there is a much greater feeling of working together at all levels. It used to be quite separate, used to operate in silos—education and practice'.

The other key advantage was undertaking the pilot as part of collaborative research because this was seen as effective and had benefits for education (CPIT) as well as informing the project group. It was seen as a positive process whereby we could adapt the model to the Canterbury setting. On completion of the pilot and evaluation, the governance group and the Canterbury Directors of Nursing (DONs), including hospital, primary and community DONs, made the formal decision that the DEU was the preferred model for clinical placements. Following the pilot period and when looking to establish further DEUs, one of the key advantages that the CNMs identified was staff recruitment, in particular for new graduates. The ability of the DEU to adapt to meet the practice setting needs has also proven positive, as in the examples of the Nurse Maude model for community nursing and the small rural hospital being a DEU site (Ashburton Hospital).

Mary commented that before the DEU model was introduced, both education and practice wanted 'to make it better' than the then current situation. A considerable advantage was the effective engagement by staff at CPIT and the DHB who had support from the nurse leaders from both organisations. Release time for the new CLN role and who was going to pay for it were some of the issues. This was an internal issue for the DHB but it signifies how 'fixed' or small issues can derail good initiatives. The budget and staying within it was by far the greatest barrier, even though the cost was very little. Mary stated, 'There was no concept that we (CDHB) were being paid to have students on clinical placement and that this money was the obvious source to cover the release time, as it was not obvious to the CNM or their immediate managers'. This barrier was removed by the Executive DON covering the release time.

One of the key areas that has not picked up the model is primary care, which seems to be in the environment of small general practice businesses. But, as

Cathy stated, 'I am struggling to think of any disadvantages of the DEU model. It better meets workforce needs, enhances relationships and anecdotally helps improve student retention in the programme'. We have exceeded our estimation that we would have 20 DEUs within five years of starting. We currently have 18 DEU practice areas within the Canterbury Health Service, only three years on from the DEU pilot project (2007). We have DEUs in the acute tertiary setting, elective hospital, rehabilitation, Older Persons—Assessment, Treatment and Rehabilitation—and Specialist Mental Health. We have also established a community nursing DEU and a small hospital DEU.

We are nearly getting to capacity and manageability and have identified the model is not for every area. The evaluation is ongoing. It is exciting to have links with other areas to find out what the common challenges and issues are. When people first hear of the DEU they think of it as a physical entity, rather than a set of principles. The future will continue to evolve and change, but the DEU is the foreseeable model of choice and we hope to extend to as many clinical areas as appropriate. We have the challenge of incorporating the impact of the new Enrolled Nurse (EN) programme within the existing DEUs and also integrating the newly qualified RNs undertaking the Nursing Entry to Practice Programmes. It may be that the DEU model may not exist in the future in the form it does now.

Members of the WG are discussing the expansion of the DEU model with other health professionals such as medical and allied health staff. The other key component would be to develop further research opportunities within the DEU model.

'One of the major successes of the DEU model within Canterbury has been the change of attitude towards student nurses by the practice environment, and the development of positive relationships between practice and education', said Mary. 'There have been significant gains for nursing within Canterbury. It has also raised the profile of nursing within the broad governance framework, and profiled nursing as a proactive profession who address issues and are proactive in workforce development'.

The DEU is an opportunity for staff development, particularly in clinical. It has given the RN an opportunity to see if it is the right time to seek promotion. As Cathy commented, 'Working together in terms of commitment to clinical learning has been beneficial for all parties at both organisational and individual levels'.

Conclusion

Regardless of an individual's role in a DEU or the clinical context of their DEU, the reflective experiences recounted in this chapter enforce the critical elements within DEUs: students and clinical and academic staff working together as a team of learners, nurses and educators; students' extended period of time in DEUs facilitating the development of strong collegial, personal and professional relationships and time to practise; ongoing feedback and assessment; strong University-health service organisation partnerships; and clinical and academic staff capacity building to add value for the staff and sustainability for the DEUs.

Above all, the stories demonstrate one of the key actions identified for developing and implementing DEUs; they have shared with a wide audience the DEU concept and knowledge about how it works (see Edgecombe et al., Chap. 11, this volume).

Reference

ANMC (n.d.). *ANMC competencies*. Australian Nursing and Midwifery Council. http://www.nursingmidwiferyboard.gov.au/Codes-Guidelines-Statements/Codes-Guidelines.aspx. Accessed 16 Aug 2012.

Chapter 11
From Conceptualisation to Future Expansion: Keys to Successful Dedicated Education Unit Implementation and Sustainability

Kay Edgecombe, Judith (Judy) Gonda, and Margaret Bowden

Glossary of Terms in Order of Appearance in This Chapter

Christchurch Polytechnic Institute of Technology/Canterbury District Health Board partnership CPIT/CDHB

Clinical Lecturer   academic staff in non-DEU clinical learning models who visit the clinical learning setting intermittently to provide curriculum integration and monitor the student's progress with the student and their preceptor; may also undertake research projects in the clinical setting

Clinical Liaison Nurse (CLN)   an experienced Registered Nurse (RN) selected from the practice area who takes on extra responsibilities, including overseeing clinical learning in the DEU and liaising between staff, students and academics/faculty (particularly the ALN); the liaison between the unit and the University; equivalent role to the DLN (University of Canberra DEUs) and LN (Flinders University DEUs)

Academic Liaison Nurse (ALN)   a permanent clinical lecturer at the University who provides consistent support to students and clinicians

Principal Academic (PA)   an academic lecturer in clinical (nursing school faculty member) who visits the clinical setting prior to student placement to facilitate clinical staff preparation for working with the students, and thereafter

K. Edgecombe (✉) • M. Bowden
School of Nursing and Midwifery, Flinders University, GPO Box 2100, Adelaide, South Australia, Australia, 5001
e-mail: kay.edgecombe@flinders.edu.au; margaret.bowden@internode.on.net; margaret.bowden@flinders.edu.au

J. (Judy) Gonda
Faculty of Health Sciences, Australian Catholic University, Brisbane, QLD, Australia
e-mail: Judith.Gonda@acu.edu.au

K. Edgecombe and M. Bowden (eds.), *Clinical Learning and Teaching Innovations in Nursing*, Innovation and Change in Professional Education 10,
DOI 10.1007/978-94-007-7232-8_11,

visits the clinical setting regularly throughout each semester; communicates and liaises with students, the CLN/DLN/LN and the CNC, and utilises their ongoing expertise to facilitate students' learning

Clinical Nurse Consultant (CNC) in charge of the ward in which the DEU operates

Registered Nurse (RN) College or University qualified nurse licensed by a nursing registration body to undertake all facets of nursing in accordance with the body's regulations

Charge Nurse Manager (CNM) takes responsibility for 'appointing' a RN to the Clinical Liaison Role (CLN), and rostering time for preparation, orientation and assessment as well as attendance at staff development/capacity building sessions

Nursing Council of New Zealand NCNZ

Introduction

Doing a Dedicated Education Unit (DEU) involves a shift of mind-set at all levels of the University and the partnering health care service organisations. Implementing a new strategy for clinical education necessarily involves cultural change, which encompasses changes in curriculum, pedagogy, roles and responsibilities and management systems (including administration, research, evaluation for quality assurance, risk mitigation and marketing). A willingness to consider and test new concepts is essential.

Conceptualisation

Frustration with the status quo was the impetus for the initial DEU concept, which developed from an integrative and equal partnership between:

- Practical experience (academic and clinical)
- Pedagogical theory
- Research (into others' experiences)

The concept (see Edgecombe, Chap. 2, this volume) was grounded solidly in many years of experience in nursing practice and academia, adult learning theory, discussion with academic teachers, clinical staff and students and research into the literature to assess the issues that continually arose in relation to nursing students' practice learning, particularly since the shift from hospital-based only to

Table 11.1 CPIT/CDHB comparison between their preceptorship and DEU clinical education models

Preceptorship model	DEU model
No dedicated on-site support person	CLN(s) identified for each DEU
Lack of consistent Clinical Lecturer (CL)	Consistent ALN who becomes familiar with the DEU practice area
CL and preceptor responsible for student orientation	ALN and CLN responsible for student orientation (supernumerary time provided for the CLN)
Individual preceptors responsible for facilitating the students learning	All DEU staff responsible for facilitating student learning
Clinical assessment completed by the preceptor and CL	Clinical assessment completed by CLN and ALN with staff input (supernumerary time provided for the CLN)
Some CDHB staff unfamiliar with BN curriculum	CLN and DEU staff are familiar with BN curriculum
Students are responsible for their own learning	Students are responsible for their own learning
	CLN coordinates student learning on a day-to-day basis
	CLN is supported by the ALN/CPIT Course Leader
	CLN provides on-site, consistent and accessible support to students and staff
	Student peer teaching encouraged
	ALN is able to offer on-site teaching sessions/research support to staff and students
1–2 students per ward/unit	Increased student numbers. Minimum six per DEU
CL allocated several students across the CDHB; therefore duty hours allocated to the CL spread across clinical areas	Contact hours for the ALN are consolidated so that the ALN is able to spend increased time in the DEU. More students = more ALN support

Source: Jamieson et al. (2008). *Establishing Dedicated Education Units for Undergraduate Nursing Students: Pilot Project Summation Report*. CPIT Publishing: New Zealand, p. 8. Used with permission from the authors and CPIT/CDHB

joint University and hospital-based teaching and learning in the 1990s. Concerns about a theory-practice gap abounded. Despite implementing different models of student nurse education, nursing as a profession was dogged by the perception of inadequate integration of theory and practice. The new way of providing nurse education demanded a new approach to students' learning in the clinical setting to facilitate higher levels of theory-practice integration, not only for students but also for academic and clinical staff. This new approach, the DEU, also addressed the issue of increased demand for nursing student clinical placements at a time of shortage of placement venues.

Since the inception of the first DEU at Flinders University, other universities who have adopted it and adapted it to suit their context-specific needs have followed a similar conceptual process, as described in Chaps. 4, 5, 6, 7 and 8 (this volume). The CPIT/CDHBcomparison between their preceptorship and DEU models is provided here to highlight the DEU's perceived and real benefits in practice for students and clinical and academic staff (Table 11.1).

Laying the Foundations

Sharing the Concept

The first step in laying the foundations for the DEU is to have the courage to stand by the concept and take the lead in sharing it with academics and clinical staff for initial feedback, then with the wider academic community in Schools of Nursing, leaders of health service organisations with whom the Schools already have practice learning partnerships, clinical staff and other potential clinical partners. Targeting potential partners who would be most willing to try the DEU concept is an important part of this dissemination and marketing process.

It is essential to explain clearly the DEU's principles, purpose, context (University and clinical settings), nature of the integration of University and practice-based people and knowledge, curriculum issues, the learning (pedagogy), partnerships and supports that will be available to all stakeholders (adapted from Cooper et al. 2010). This includes clearly defined roles and responsibilities, management processes and lines of communication.

Holding meetings for discussion, debate and to seek further partners results in a core group of stakeholders who can see the potential benefits of the DEU. They are *willing to take the risk* and a leadership role in putting the shared concept into practice. Each leader will have 'an appreciation for how the DEU concept complements their vision for their departments and for nursing as a profession' (Glazer et al. 2011). Marketing the DEU concept can involve making use of already established strong personal relationships and University-health service organisation relationships, face-to-face meetings and technological tools such as videoconferences, emails and websites. The CPIT/CDHB model provides an example of marketing the DEU essentially as a collaborative model of clinical teaching and learning that:

- Facilitates a closer working relationship between CPIT nursing staff and CDHB clinical staff
- Provides consistent clinical support for students
- Increases understanding of BN curriculum amongst clinical staff
- Focuses on the learning needs of students
- Encourages and values peer teaching (Casey and Whittle 2009)

Establishing Partnerships

Partnerships' contextual environments (from a systemic and organisational perspective) must be considered before approaching potential partners because, as Judy Gonda found in her research about partnerships in clinical education for nurses (Gonda 2008), organisations driven solely by cost containment and increased efficiencies are unsuitable for DEU partnerships. In assessing potential partners, you need to consider organisational characteristics such as 'geography', whether it is a 'learning organisation', its 'teaching mission', 'service lines' and 'administrative support' (Parker and Smith 2012: E3). Unit characteristics including 'leadership', 'intraprofessional collaboration', 'teamwork', 'communication', 'resources' and 'cultural diversity' (Parker and Smith 2012: E3) also require consideration. Parker and Smith (2012: E3) identify nursing practice ('differentiated practice', 'maturity of the unit' and 'shared governance') as an additional group of structural factors for consideration in assessing a unit's suitability for a DEU. However, partnership is always a two-way street, and potential partners will want to know what the benefits are for them. The American Association of Colleges of Nursing (AACN 2010) has developed some useful resources for setting up and evaluating academic-practice partnerships.

Partnership Levels

It is also essential to remember when establishing partnerships that these involve several partnership levels. First, partnerships must be established at the higher organisational levels of health service organisations (boards and CEOs) and universities (Vice-Chancellors and Heads of Schools of Nursing) to ensure the policies, procedures and financial and administrative resources that are put in place will result in success (Gonda 2008). In addition, there must be willingness at this level to support the introduction of DEUs.

Once a partnership agreement has been reached at the organisational level, the next step is to establish partnerships between the University and the Heads of Nursing, the University and the Heads of wards/units (e.g. Clinical Nurse Consultants—CNCs). Other levels of partnership necessary for DEUs to function successfully lie with the relationships between the Heads of Nursing, Heads of wards/units, ward/unit staff, students and clinical facilitators. DEU partnerships require all stakeholders to adopt a leadership role in participating in what is essentially a clinical learning and teaching community of practice, as described by Grealish et al. (Chap. 3, this volume). Underlying each leader's interest will be 'an appreciation for how the DEU concept complements their vision for their departments and for nursing as a profession' (Glazer et al. 2011).

Members at the higher levels of the partnership hierarchy need to solicit and seriously consider the views of other stakeholders in the DEU who will be affected by particular decisions before acting on them. Consequences of these decisions need to be evaluated, analysed and reported to all stakeholders continuously in an informal manner and as a formal process in the early stages of the partnership (Gonda 2008).

Equal, Committed, Enduring Investment and Value

Principal Academics (PAs), CNCs and RNs are supported in their roles through strategies that ensure equal, committed and *enduring* investment, such as realistically adjusted workloads and capacity building/staff development, and recognition and reward in the form of professional awards and promotion (Gonda 2008). Valuing all partners equally means they have a say in decisions that involve implementing the DEU in particular health care contexts and work together continuously towards achieving the mutually agreed goals of the DEU. The CPIT/CDHB DEU exemplifies the ingredients for a successful partnership. We use it in the next section as an illustration of how to do a DEU.

Implementation: 'Doing a DEU'

Piloting the Concept

Once the partnerships between the University and the health service organisation have been established, the first step in implementing the DEU involves piloting the concept. The pilot and subsequent DEUs require ongoing cycles of planning, preparation, action (implementation), evaluation (research), renovation and marketing (including face-to-face meetings, forums, website, newsletters, brochures and reports). An important part of the pilot stage is consultation with a critical friend who has experience of DEUs and can be called upon for support throughout the DEU implementation and embedding stages. The CPIT/CDHB visited Flinders University School of Nursing DEU academic staff who acted in this role.

Setting up a Steering Committee or Governance Group is recommended as a good practice strategy for providing advice to the pilot project team and overseeing the project's implementation. The following illustrations demonstrate the CPIT/CDHB Governance model (Fig. 11.1), and the partnership, group and support structures set up to pilot the DEU in Christchurch, New Zealand (Fig. 11.2).

Recruitment

Recruitment of a pilot clinical site, academics and students can be done through applications/expressions of interest to ensure a high participation rate amongst those who are interested and willing. This is also a competitive process.

Preparation

It is essential to prepare the clinical setting (in particular the clinicians), students and academics. Preparation of clinicians can involve information at informal and formal staff meetings at work and orientation workshops at the University to give them an overview of the DEU concept, an introduction to teaching/learning theory and some clinical teaching strategies. Students can be prepared through

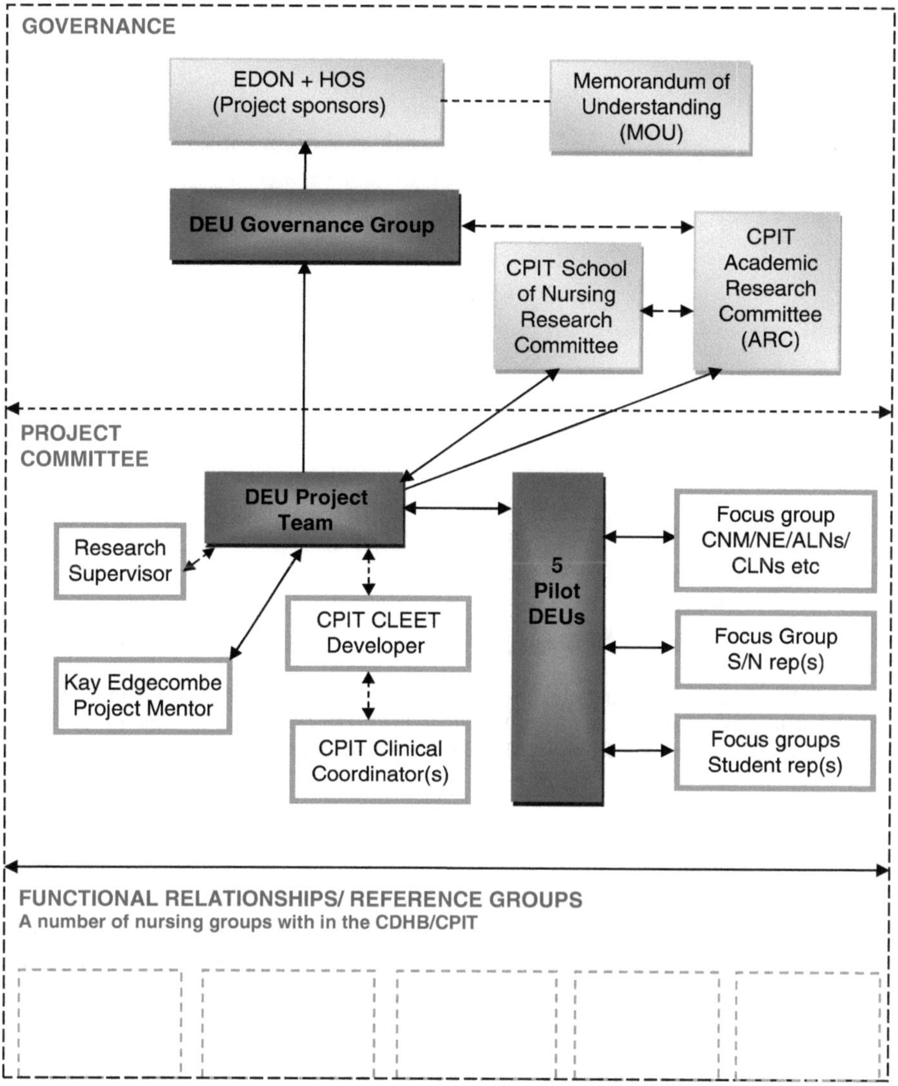

Fig. 11.1 CPIT DEU governance model (Used with permission from Michelle Casey (CDHB), Deb Sims (CPIT) and the CDHB/CPIT DEU Governance and Working Groups)

meetings at which they receive an overview of the DEU concept, shift requirements and start and completion dates, as well as thorough orientation to the DEU clinical environment. Similarly, academics can be prepared through workshops and meetings with the clinicians. It is essential that all have a solid understanding of what drives the DEU and how this strategy differs from other clinical education strategies.

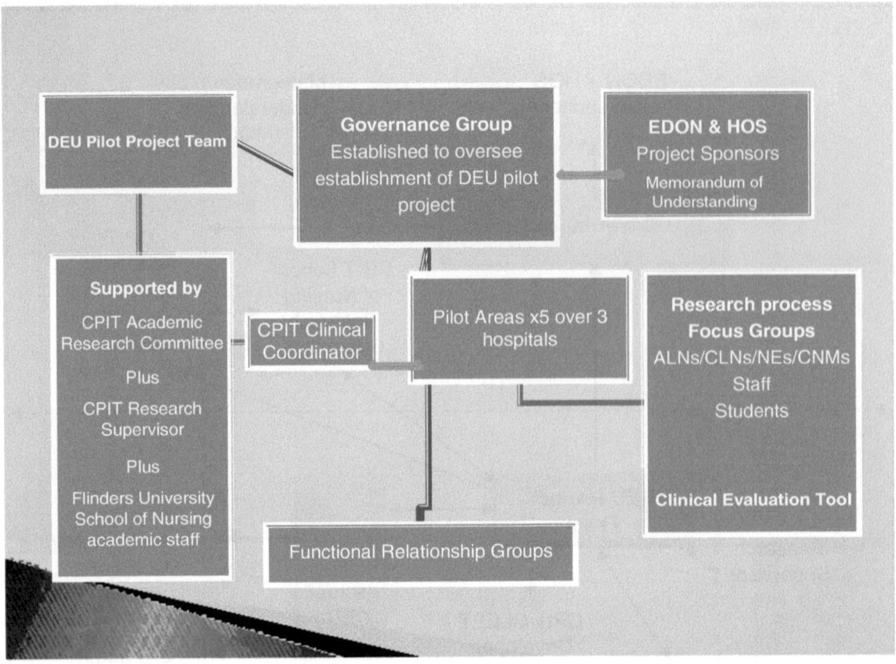

Fig. 11.2 Partnership, group and support structures for piloting the DEU. Used with permission from Michelle Casey (CDHB) and Rose Whittle (CPIT), *The Dedicated Education Unit (DEU) model of clinical teaching and learning*, May 2009 (powerpoint presentation)

Visualisation

Providing a visual model of the DEU during the preparation stage can help participants understand the collaborative relationships amongst them. The CPIT/CDHB graphic is used here as an illustration of the type of visualisation needed (Fig. 11.3). Providing a comparison with the model/s currently in use can further enhance participants' understanding of the DEU and its points of difference (Fig. 11.4).

Roles and Responsibilities

Understanding new roles and responsibilities is paramount for those participating in the DEU pilot. These will be explained during preparation sessions but will also evolve during the pilot. It is crucial that sufficient support is provided to enable those undertaking specific roles (e.g. the CLN or the ALN) to perform their roles to the level required to meet the DEU's objectives. In the CPIT/CDHB DEUs, the CLN role incorporates specific DEU time allocations. These consist of 8 h away from the ward/unit to attend a DEU workshop, 8 h per student

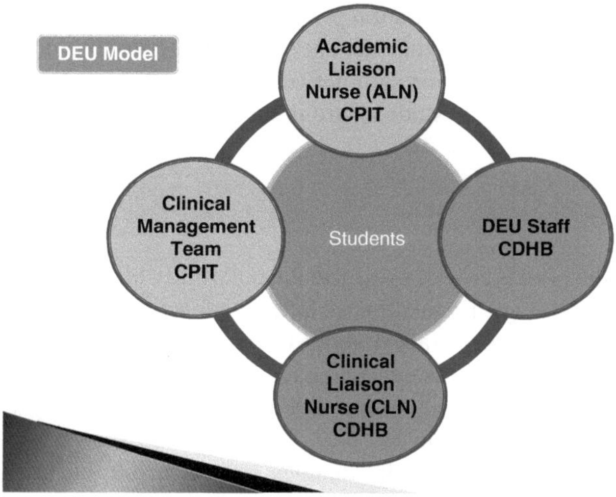

Fig. 11.3 CPIT/CDHB DEU model. Used with permission from Michelle Casey (CDHB) and Rose Whittle (CPIT), *The Dedicated Education Unit (DEU) model of clinical teaching and learning*, May 2009 (powerpoint presentation)

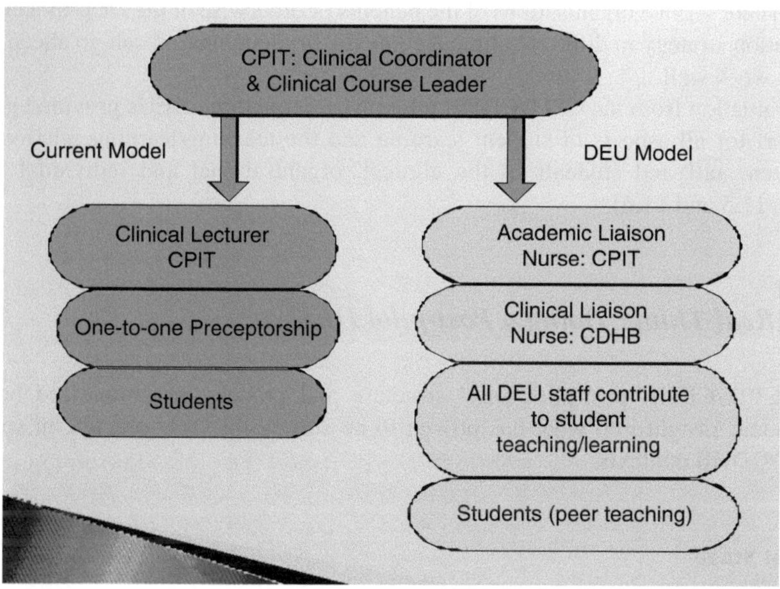

Fig. 11.4 DEU compared to current model. Used with permission from Michelle Casey (CDHB) and Rose Whittle (CPIT), *The Dedicated Education Unit (DEU) model of clinical teaching and learning*, May 2009 (powerpoint presentation)

placement administration/preparation prior to students arriving in the ward/unit, 8 h for orientation activities with students, one and a half hours per student for formative assessment, 1 h per student for summative assessment and half an hour daily for CLN-related activities while students are in the ward/unit.

Evaluation

Evaluation of the pilot is crucial to inform the possibility of implementing DEUs as a clinical learning strategy. Evaluation includes feedback from all those participating in the pilot. It covers issues raised about time, roles, workload, support, teaching and learning (including assessment), curriculum, administration, cost, recognition and reward. Above all, it needs to measure the real outcomes against the intended outcomes of the DEU: *Will it work?*

Acting on the initial feedback, changes can be made and a renovated DEU implemented as an extended or second pilot to ensure thorough testing before full implementation. The second/extended pilot can test new roles and suggested changes from the initial pilot. This is essential to ensure successful implementation of the DEU if it is decided to adopt it.

Further feedback from the second/extended pilot will inform universities and health care service organisations of the benefits or otherwise of the DEU as a clinical education strategy in different clinical contexts. Implementation can go ahead if the pilots work well.

Evaluation from the CPIT/CDHB pilot project found the DEUs provided greater support for all aspects of student learning and the teaching/learning relationships between staff and students at the clinical, organisational and individual levels (Figs. 11.5 and 11.6).

The Real Thing: Doing a Post-pilot DEU

The CPIT/CDHB post-pilot DEU structure and process is summarised here to give clear insight into what has proven to be successful DEU practice in specific CPIT/CDHB contexts.

Initial Stage

1. Articulate a shared philosophy between the University (CPIT) and its health services organisation partner (CDHB)—document and disseminate.
2. Agree on where to establish DEUs.
3. Articulate the principles underpinning the partnership between CPIT School of Nursing and the DEU practice area—document and disseminate to all partners and potential partners.

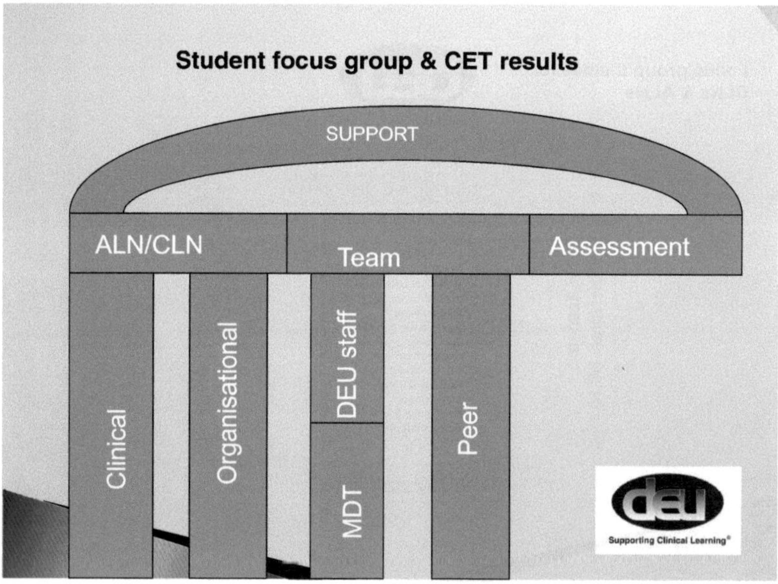

Fig. 11.5 Student evaluation re teaching and learning support in DEU. Used with permission from Michelle Casey (CDHB) and Rose Whittle (CPIT), *The Dedicated Education Unit (DEU) model of clinical teaching and learning*, May 2009 (powerpoint presentation)

4. Establish a management structure, beginning with a DEU Working Group (had previously been the Pilot Project Team) to maintain and develop the DEU model of clinical teaching and learning within Canterbury DHB venues (Fig. 11.7).
5. Establish a Governance Group to provide guidance to the Working Group (members of the Working Group are also members of the Governance Group).
6. Clearly outline, document and disseminate the terms of reference for both groups, as per the CPIT/CDHB examples on the following pages.
7. Second, a Nurse Educator (an original member of the Working Group) to support implementation of additional DEUs. The Nurse Educator works closely with DEU staff and the CPIT clinical management team and represents the CDHB on CPIT committees.
8. Clearly outline, document and disseminate roles and responsibilities of DEU participants, for example, Clinical Liaison Nurse (CLN), Academic Liaison Nurse (ALN), DEU staff (including RNs, ENs, Nurse Assistants, pool nurses and Medical and Allied Health staff) and students (Fig. 11.8).
9. Clearly outline, document and disseminate requirements for application for particular roles, for example, for the CLN role (Fig. 11.9).
10. Incorporate DEU principles when recruiting staff in DEU practice areas.
11. Provide training for new CLNs, ALNs, CNMs and key nursing staff via workshops each semester.

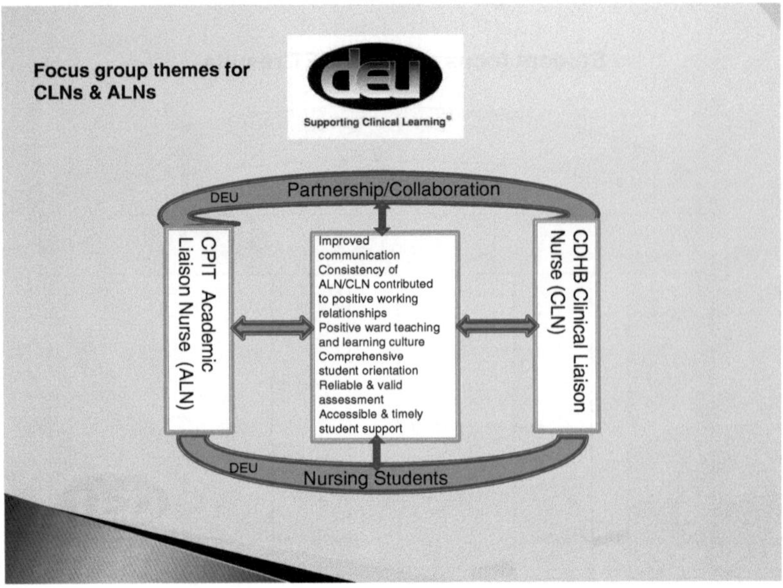

Fig. 11.6 CLN and ALN evaluation re teaching and learning support in DEU. Used with permission from Michelle Casey (CDHB) and Rose Whittle (CPIT), *The Dedicated Education Unit (DEU) model of clinical teaching and learning*, May 2009 (powerpoint presentation)

12. Clearly outline number of students for each DEU based on individual DEU skill mix and Full Time Equivalents and DEU bed numbers, with a minimum of three students per shift. Also identify required learning opportunities, including Skill repetition, One-to-one teaching, Peer teaching, Incidental learning and Diversity of learning.
13. Implement use of communications tools, such as the Clinical Practice Diary to assist with communication between staff and between students and staff. This is an ongoing assessment tool as well as maintaining lines of communication. We provide a sample of a Clinical Practice Diary in Fig. 11.10.

Establishment Stage: DEU Embedded, Sustainable and Looking Forward

Once the initial DEU has been operating successfully for several semesters, it can be considered to be established. Understanding when the establishment or embedded stage has been reached depends on evaluation of the initial implementation stage, and the DEU's ability to run effectively with reduced input from the initial Working Party; it has become sustainable in its current context and should now have the ability to flex and change as the contextual environment changes.

CPIT

Canterbury
District Health Board
Te Poari Hauora ō Waitaha

Terms of Reference

Dedicated Education Unit Working Group

April 2009

Scope	The DEU Working Group will oversee the day-to-day running of existing DEU's and actively promote and develop the DEU model of Clinical Teaching and Learning in interested practice areas within the CDHB
Purpose	For CPIT and CDHB to maintain and develop the Dedicated Education Unit model of clinical teaching and learning within Canterbury DHB
Objectives	1. To ensure existing DEU's are maintained and reflect Canterbury DEU models philosophy 2. To support the establishment of new DEUs 3. To provide leadership and support to the staff and students in the DEU practice areas 4. To continue to work collaboratively with CPIT and CDHB staff 5. To continue to monitor the DEU practice areas 6. To report to the Governance Group on: monitoring outcomes 7. To develop and implement action plans as agreed to by the Governance Group
Accountability	The DEU Working Group is accountable to the DEU Governance Group
Membership	• Two Nurse Educators, CDHB • Two Nurse Lectures, CPIT • Clinical Manager, CPIT • Undergraduate nursing student coordinator, CDHB • Each member to be appointed for a two-year term with the right of renewal
Co-chairpersons	• Clinical Manager, CPIT • Undergraduate nursing student coordinator, CDHB
Quorum	Majority
Meetings	Fortnightly and as required
Agenda	Circulate 3 days prior to meeting
Minutes	Circulate within 1 week following meeting and confirmation of minutes to occur at next meeting
Decision making	Wherever possible by consensus. If unable to concur, then decision will be by majority vote
Functional relationships with other groups and committees	Governance Group DEU Charge Nurse Managers CPIT Clinical and Academic Managers
Communications responsibilities	
Appointment process	The Executive Director of Nursing, CDHB and the Nursing Head of School, CPIT will be responsible to appoint appropriate members to the DEU Working Group as per the membership section of this document
Resignation process	Members are required to submit their resignation to the Governance Group in writing providing at least one month's notice
New members	New members will be orientated to DEU Working Group by a member of the working group
Review of terms of reference	These Terms of Reference will be reviewed by the DEU Working Group yearly

Fig. 11.7 DEU working group terms of reference (Used with permission of CPIT and CDHB)

CPIT Canterbury District Health Board Te Poari Hauora ō Waitaha

Terms of Reference

Dedicated Education Unit Governance Group

June 2009

Scope	The Dedicated Education Unit (DEU) Governance Group (GG) is a decision-making group with a mandate to oversee the maintenance of current DEU practice areas and to assist the DEU Working Group in the establishment of the DEU model to interested practice areas within Canterbury District Health Board (CDHB)
Purpose	To monitor, approve, resource and oversee the establishment, maintenance and evaluation of DEUs within the CDHB
Objectives	1. To provide guidance, support and direction to the DEU Working Group 2. To ensure current DEUs are monitored and new DEUs are supported 3. To oversee the evaluation of all DEUs 4. To provide leadership and support to the DEU practice areas 5. To develop a strategic research plan for DEUs
Accountability	The GG is accountable to the Executive Director of Nursing, CDHB and the Head of School: School of Nursing and Human Services, Christchurch Polytechnic Institute of Technology (CPIT)
Membership	• Executive Director of Nursing: CDHB • Head of School: School of Nursing and Human Services, CPIT • A nominated Divisional Director of Nursing: CDHB • A nominated member of the Nurse Entry to Practice Programme (NETP): CDHB • Clinical Manager: School of Nursing, CPIT • Nurse Coordinator—Preregistration Nursing Students Role: CDHB (Currently seconded Nurse Educator, DEU) • DEU Working Group members • Nursing Leaders: Primary/Community
Chairperson	Executive Director of Nursing: CDHB
Co-chairperson	Head of School: School of Nursing and Human Services, CPIT
Quorum	50% plus chair
Meetings	Monthly, 1530–1700 hours, 3rd Thursday of the month
Agenda	Circulate 3 days prior to meeting
Minutes	Circulate minutes to GG members and to the Directors of Nursing. Circulate within 1 week following meeting and confirmation of minutes to occur at next meeting
Subgroup	Subgroups may be established by the GG to activate and/or co-ordinate specific work/tasks as seen fit by the GG. All subgroups will be adequately briefed by the GG and resourced to enable full achievement of the tasks/work assigned At least one (1) Governance Group member will be part of any subgroup established
Decision making	Consensus with equal representation from each organisation
Functional relationships with other groups and committees	• Canterbury District Health Board Directors of Nursing (DONs) Group • CDHB NETP Group • Clinical Practice Committee, CPIT • Southern Region Nurse Executives New Zealand (NENZ) • CPIT School of Nursing Advisory Committee
Communications responsibilities	Communication will occur in partnership across both organisations, recognising the collaborative nature of DEUs
Review of terms of reference	These terms of reference will be reviewed by the Governance Group annually

Fig. 11.8 DEU governance group terms of reference (Used with permission of CPIT and CDHB)

E Tauratia Nga Akoranga Hauora Putaiao

Supporting Clinical Learning®

Checklist for Appointment to Clinical Liaison Nurse (CLN) Role

The Nursing Leader appointing the CLN and the Registered Nurse complete this form together using the tick box and writing comments in the boxes provided. If role is to be shared, please complete a separate form for each individual.

RN Name:	Practice Area:	Tick box	Name of Nursing Leader (NL):
Had Performance Review within last year?			Date:
Are they on PDRP programme?			Competent/ Proficient/ Expert *Please circle relevant one*
Has RN read CLN Roles and Responsibilities on the CDHB intranet or Internet?			*CDHB Internet—CLN role* *www.cdhb.govt.nz/deu/default.htm*
Had discussion with NL about CLN role, DEU model and workplace contribution etc.			
Had discussion with NL regarding impact of annual leave/ study leave/ commitments during student placements?			
Does RN have regular access to a workplace computer?			Access to a computer is essential
Does RN have a CDHB email address?			*If you do not have one, this will be arranged*
Please provide your email address			
RN can be contacted on the following phone numbers:			Ward ext: Cellphone:
Comments/Other Requirements:			
*Name of RN:*_______________________ *appointed to* CLN role for the DEU model in the practice area Date:			NL Signature:
I (*Name of RN*)________________________ accept appointment of CLN Role for the DEU model in the practice area. Date:			CLN Signature:
Please keep a copy for yourself and fax or send a copy of the checklist to Name, CDHB Nurse Educator DEU DEU name Ph: xxx-xxxx Fax: xxx-xxxx (External) xxxxx (Internal)			Date:

cc. Nurses personal file

Fig. 11.9 CPIT/CDHB checklist for appointment to clinical liaison nurse role (Used with permission of CPIT and CDHB)

CPIT/CDHB Clinical Practice Diary

Student Name________________________ Clinical Area____________ Clinical Lecturer________________________

Please use this to keep a daily diary of activities and significant experiences you feel will help you and the staff evaluate your daily performance
Areas for Possible Focus : - Communication skills - Time management skills - Holistic assessment skills - Nursing care plans - Documentation - Clinical skill performance - Team work - Participation in learning opportunities - Knowledge of drugs/safe drug administration practice - Ability to provide rationale for nursing actions - Linking theory to practice

Student Daily Focus and Activities/Review of day	Brief Comment from Allocated Nurse: Suggested Focus for Next Shift
Monday Date: Focus: Review of Day:	What the Student Did well: Suggested Focus for Next Shift: Nurse Initials:
Tuesday Date: Focus: Review of Day:	What the Student Did well: Suggested Focus for Next Shift: Nurse Initials:
Wednesday Date: Focus: Review of Day:	What the Student Did well: Suggested Focus for Next Shift: Nurse Initials:
Thursday Date: Focus: Review of Day:	What the Student Did well: Suggested Focus for Next Shift: Nurse Initials:
Friday Date: Focus: Review of Day:	What the Student Did well: Suggested Focus for Next Shift: Nurse Initials:

Fig. 11.10 CPIT/CDHB clinical practice diary (Used with permission from CPIT/CDHB)

deu

E Tauràtia Ngā Akoranga Hauora Pūtaiao

Supporting Clinical Learning®

Certificate of Recognition

This certificate is presented to the staff of

Ward 28

to acknowledge their commitment to the DEU model of clinical teaching and learning with nursing students in the Canterbury health system.
A Dedicated Education Unit (DEU) is a practice area dedicated to supporting undergraduate nursing students.

Awarded on 30 July 2010

Canterbury District Health Board Te Poari Hauora o Waitaha

Mary Gordon,
Executive Director of Nursing,
CDHB
Te Poari Hauora o Waitaha

Cathy Andrew,
Head of School, Nursing & Human Services,
CPIT

CPIT

Fig. 11.11 Proposed certificate of recognition for the ward/unit (Used with permission from CDHB/CPIT)

Key strategies during the establishment stage to engender engagement and a sense of belonging amongst organisations, staff and students participating in DEUs, as well as continuing to market the DEU and build expansion and sustainability, include:

1. Recognition and reward, for example, a DEU certificate for the ward/unit (see Fig. 11.11).

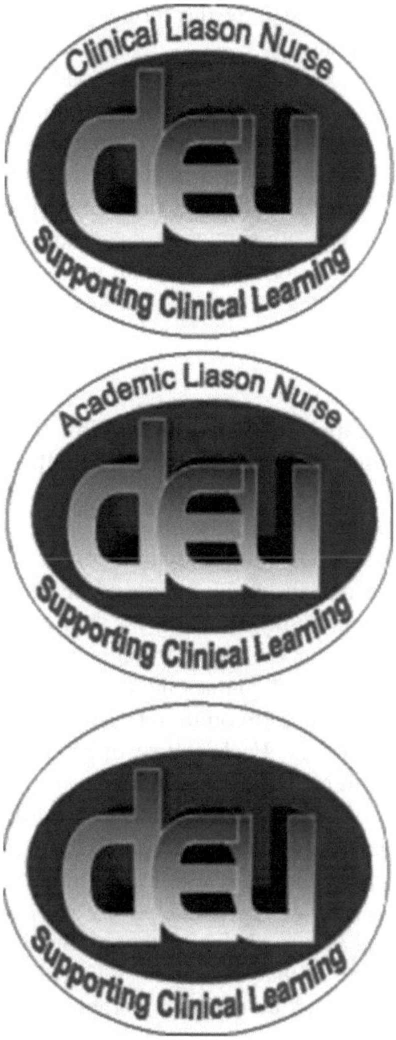

Fig. 11.12 Example of badges for DEU participants (Used with permission from CDHB/CPIT)

2. Badges for DEU participants (see Fig. 11.12), which give a sense of belonging to the DEU.
3. Ongoing evaluation/audit of the DEU via feedback from all participants.
4. Ongoing quality maintenance involving all participants, including a 5-yearly review. Strategies, as outlined by Casey et al. (Chap. 7, this volume), include face-to-face evaluation meetings, DEU key indicators, an audit planner, a review of DEU documents (includes Philosophy, Roles and Responsibilities), an annual DEU Workshop, support for existing DEUs (includes updating intranet and Internet), ongoing promotion of the model (includes updating information brochure and website), ongoing maintenance of the model and support from the DEU Governance Group.

5. Planning for the future—develop a strategic plan (CPIT/CDHB has a five-year plan).
6. Seeking new directions and possibilities for DEUs in different contexts—new partnerships, research and innovation.
7. Constant local and global dissemination of the DEU and resources for setting up new DEUs in different contexts via the Internet (http://www.cdhb.govt.nz/deu/default.htm), publications, conference presentations, face-to-face meetings with other interested Schools of Nursing and health service organisations, and collaborative research and publication with others already using the DEU as a strategy to address clinical learning and teaching issues and nursing workforce issues.

Clear Demonstration of How the DEU Fits Within the Structure of Clinical Placements Across the CPIT Bachelor of Nursing Degree Programme

The CPIT Bachelor of Nursing (BN) is a 3-year undergraduate programme, providing students with theoretical and clinical courses. The curriculum is designed to meet the requirements of the Nursing Council of New Zealand (NCNZ) Education Programme Standards for the Registered Nurse Scope of Practice (NCNZ 2005) and the Competencies for Registered Nurses (NCNZ 2007).

Clinical courses include a range of practice experiences that must occur in both hospital and community settings. Students bear the costs for access to healthcare providers. Each course offers minimum and maximum clinical hours, consistent with NCNZ requirements.

The NCNZ registers successful graduates as Registered Nurses (RNs). Clinical lecturers employed by CPIT, in conjunction with RNs employed in the specific clinical area, assess the learning outcomes and competencies, based on the NCNZ competencies. Students are expected to demonstrate an increase in independent behaviour related to the application of knowledge, skills and attitudes over the 3 years of the programme. Clinical practice placements across the 3-year levels follow the structure outlined in Table 11.2.

Conclusion

Dedicated Education Units can take different forms depending on the clinical, organisational and education outcomes contexts in which they are implemented. The example of the successful CPIT/CDHB processes for planning, piloting and implementing their DEUs encompasses all the elements of DEUs described in other chapters in this book. It places additional emphasis on marketing and staff identification strategies, particularly having DEU staff and students wear badges, which generates a sense of pride, identity and belonging.

Table 11.2 Structure of clinical placements across the 3-year undergraduate programme

Part A (Semester 1)	Part B (Semester 2)
Year 1	
Students are allocated to each clinical placement in groups of six to eight and have a clinical lecturer present for all their shifts. Clinical practice placements take place in Continuing Care settings, which have a mostly older adult population who require different levels of care ranging from assisted independent living to hospital level care	
Part A (Semester 1)	*Part B (Semester 2)*
Three half-day visits to placements to meet and introduce themselves to their allocated patients/residents, with a primary focus on communication skills as a beginning health professional	Progress to working 14 full 8-h clinical days, which mostly occur in a clinical block. Focus on developing clinical nursing and health assessment skills with allocated patients/residents
Year 2	
Part A (Semester 1)	*Part B (Semester 2)*
Mental Health placement in either a community or inpatient practice area. Students have 30 clinical days over a 7-week period. Most weeks are 4-day clinical weeks, with students working 8-h shifts, Monday to Friday, as rostered by placement staff. The clinical lecturer is present for the equivalent of 0.5 h per student per day, equating to approximately 2 h per student per week. The more students in a particular area, the greater amount of time the clinical lecturer is present	Medical/Surgical placement, either combined in one practice area that can provide this experience or in two different practice areas, one with a medical and one with a surgical specialty focus. Students have 45 days over a 10-week period, with a combination of 4 and 5-day weeks, and work 8-h shifts, Monday to Friday, as rostered by the placement staff. The clinical lecturer contact hour allocation is the same as the previous semester
Year 3	
Part A (Semester 1)	*Part B (Semester 2)*
Six-week (30 day) Community Health placement, for example, in an urban or rural medical practice, district nursing, child health nursing, corrections health (with criminal offenders) and public health nursing. Clinical lecturer supervision is decreased to the equivalent of 1.5 h per student per week (or 9 h over the 6-week placement)	Final placement. Students select an area of practice in which they are interested. May be influenced by future career plans or a need to consolidate or extend their skills in a particular area. Rostered shifts (including night shift and weekends if appropriate). Eight to 11-week placement, depending on the number of clinical hours the student needs to meet the NCNZ requirements. Clinical lecturer visits students for equivalent of 1 h per week over the placement block. This decreased contact reflects the expectation for the student to integrate and become part of the nursing team

While this chapter is not intended as a recipe for DEUs—no two DEUs will be identical due to localised conditions—it provides a foundation for those interested in setting up DEUs in that it summarises all steps from conceptualisation to implementation. We believe that these same steps can be used for developing and implementing interprofessional DEUs. This is an area for further research, which will need funding. Undertaking DEU evaluations has not been addressed specifically in this chapter, but different DEUs in different parts of the world will have different avenues for funding such research. In the USA, for example, the Robert Wood Johnson Foundation (http://evaluatinginnovationsinnursing.org/) provides funding for Evaluating Innovations in Nursing Education (EIN).

References

AACN. (2010). *Academic-practice partnerships*. http://www.aacn.nche.edu/leading-initiatives/academic-practice-partnerships. Accessed 28 Feb 2013.

Casey, M., & Whittle, R. (2009, May). *The Dedicated Education Unit (DEU) model of clinical teaching and learning*. PowerPoint presentation, CPIT, Christchurch

Cooper, L., Orrell, J., & Bowden, M. (2010). *Work integrated learning: A guide to effective practice*. London: Routledge.

Glazer, G., Erickson, J. I., Mylott, L., Mulready-Shick, J., & Banister, G. (2011). Partnering and leadership: Core requirements for developing a Dedicated Education Unit. *Journal of Nursing Administration, 41*(10), 401–406.

Gonda, J. W. (2008). *Impact of politics, systems and culture on the success of a clinical education partnership*. Dissertation, School of Nursing and Midwifery, The University of Queensland, Australia. http://espace.library.uq.edu.au/view/UQ:134430. Accessed 12 Oct 2011.

Jamieson, I., Hale, J., Sims, D., Casey, M., Whittle, R., & Kilkenny, T. (2008). *Establishing Dedicated Education Units for undergraduate nursing students: Pilot project summation report* (p. 8). Christchurch: CPIT Publishing Unit.

NCNZ. (2005). *Education programme standards for the registered nurse scope of practice*. Wellington: NCNZ.

NCNZ. (2007). *Competencies for registered nurses*. Wellington: NCNZ.

Parker, K. M., & Smith, C. M. (2012). Assessment and planning for a Dedicated Education Unit. *Journal for Nurses in Staff Development, 28*(11), E1–E6.

Chapter 12
Conclusion

Kay Edgecombe and Margaret Bowden

This book has traced the development and implementation of the DEU as a clinical learning and teaching environment. It has explored the DEU's conception (Chap. 2, this volume), framing within the pedagogical basis of a community of practice (Chap. 3, this volume), adaptation and uptake in Australia, the USA, New Zealand and Sweden (Chaps. 4, 5, 6, 7, and 8, this volume), inbuilt and formally structured capacity building (Chap. 9, this volume) and shared personal experiences (Chap. 10, this volume). Chapter 11 (Edgecombe et al., this volume), which has outlined how to do a DEU by giving examples of different processes used by the Christchurch Polytechnic Institute of Technology/Canterbury District Health Board (CPIT/CDHB) DEU partnership team, consolidates Chaps. 2, 3, 4, 5, 6, 7, 8, 9, and 10 (this volume). It completes the journey through DEUs by putting all the essential elements together in one chapter as a 'how to' guide.

Each chapter has emphasised the value of clinical and academic staff 'preparation' or 'staff/faculty development' (capacity building) as part of the overall DEU process. Strategies for structured and incidental capacity building in DEUs mentioned throughout the book have been consolidated in Chap. 9 (this volume), in which Edgecombe and Bowden outline workshops and discuss peer teaching and learning to illustrate how capacity building is inherent in DEUs.

The personal experience reflections in Chap. 10 (this volume), while illustrating the different experiences of people in different roles in different DEUs in different countries, all support the value of the DEU as a set of principles and an effective clinical education strategy. The stories provide evidence that the DEU has facilitated a better clinical learning environment than previously tried models in the contexts described. Importantly, the stories reiterate experiences of 'belonging' and 'being

K. Edgecombe (✉) • M. Bowden
School of Nursing and Midwifery, Flinders University, GPO Box 2100, Adelaide, South Australia, Australia, 5001
e-mail: kay.edgecombe@flinders.edu.au; margaret.bowden@internode.on.net; margaret.bowden@flinders.edu.au

K. Edgecombe and M. Bowden (eds.), *Clinical Learning and Teaching Innovations in Nursing*, Innovation and Change in Professional Education 10,
DOI 10.1007/978-94-007-7232-8_12, © Springer Science+Business Media Dordrecht 2014

valued' in the DEU environment, experiences that had been lacking in other placement environments. The experiences retold also raise seemingly negative issues that arise when implementing the DEU as a model of clinical learning in the clinical setting, for example, coping with increased numbers of students on a ward. However, the stories also illustrate how misgivings about numbers of students gave way to the realisation that having more students was beneficial in a DEU environment.

Importantly, although not stated overtly in most of the chapters, organisational transformation and cultural change, driven by strong leadership, lie at the heart of successfully introducing and implementing DEUs across different clinical contexts. The sense of a shared community, or a 'village' as Craig and Moscato call it in Chap. 6 (this volume), with both partners committed to developing, sustaining and maintaining a professional nurse's career, engenders a sense of shared responsibility and enthusiasm to share learning, develop the next generation of nurses and continue to pursue ongoing nurse education. It inspires academic staff, clinical staff and students to become part of the cycle of generation and regeneration that will sustain and expand DEUs.

Transformation and Cultural Change

This journey through DEUs in Nursing across the globe has demonstrated transformation and cultural change within University Schools of Nursing and health-care organisations. Shared recognition of the need for innovation, a shared vision about such an innovation and a willingness to take the risk to collaborate to implement it, evaluate it and ensure its sustainability through working in partnerships that give equal value to all their participants' input have enabled this change. The previous chapters in this volume highlight the same ingredients for beginning successful partnerships and transformation as those Flash et al. (2006) identify: sound organisational purpose understood and agreed by all partners; strong personal leadership, and recognition and use of internal talent; and a 'carefully crafted, adaptive strategy'. Above all, this book illustrates the necessity for, and the power of, like-minded people. Such people, as also identified by Flash et al. (2006), are the key ingredient in any transformational change.

Keys to Success

A sound set of foundational principles and willingness to participate stand out as crucial ingredients in the successful development and implementation of DEUs. Willingness must go beyond the initial passionate few advocates to the sustainable level of willingness to participate at a systemic level in dynamic environments with transient populations. The contributing authors and the literature emphasise that the key factor in a successful DEU is 'buy-in' at all levels of the partnering institutions and organisations.

Leadership at all levels, from those who have the initial idea to those in administrative and policy positions within universities and health-care services/organisations and to the clinical and academic staff in the clinical settings, promotes participation. Students, through their role as peer teachers as well as learners in the DEU environment, become leaders in engaging other students and, as evidenced in some of the stories in Chap. 10 (this volume), in engaging the clinical and academic staff. This willingness and engagement is needed on the part of those not directly involved with a particular DEU as well as those who are directly involved. One of the most important roles is that of a 'critical friend', a person who is willing to guide and support those who are in the process of setting up DEUs. The critical friend will be someone who has already set up DEUs and evaluated them and is willing to share their knowledge with others, making sure not to impose on a new DEU context a strict set of conditions that may have worked in earlier DEUs.

Dedicated Education Units already in operation have adhered to their foundational principles and incorporated strategies that have proven successful in developing, implementing and managing practice learning models, including:

- Clear purpose
- Leadership
- Communication
- Collaboration, which involves support from hospital and university management and administrative support
- Clear role and responsibility delineation
- Clear management processes
- Flexibility
- Innovation
- Evaluation
- Re-innovation (see Cooper et al. 2010; Sims 2008)

All of these elements are included in the trial stage. After evaluation, re-innovation informs the second and subsequent DEUs. Staff capacity building is a key part of the collaborative support and management processes at all stages.

Administration

Administration requires more attention. In the Introduction to this volume, we made the point that research into clinical learning models tends to overlook administration. Although we hoped to include more detail about the nuts and bolts of administration, this role tends to be implied within the terms of reference for governance groups or committees, for example, in the sample CPIT/CDHB forms provided in Chap. 11 (Edgecombe et al., this volume). However, effective administration is central to the whole DEU strategy, particularly in terms of researching and disseminating information about the roles, responsibilities and networks required to help organisations and individuals understand the DEU's administrative basis. Keeping lines of communication going, controlling computer systems and working every day to ensure everything runs smoothly are largely assumed, as is promotion and marketing. Judy Gonda (Chap. 4, this volume) places some focus on administration, as do Casey et al. (Chap. 7, this volume), which is evidenced in the CPIT/CDHB forms presented in Chap. 11 (Edgecombe et al., this volume). However, there is a need for a greater balance in focus between the vision, the how to, the doing (the teaching and learning) and the day-to-day administration, which is a rarely acknowledged part of DEU management.

There is also the quandary of how to 'sell' the DEU concept. As identified by CPIT/CDHB, the DEU is not a concrete thing. It is a set of principles on which to base various manifestations of the basic DEU model for clinical learning to fit particular contexts. The DEU's form can change to suit the context and its resources, which is a complex concept to market and understand when most models are rigid and take the same concrete form in all contexts.

Harnessing the enthusiasm of those who have experienced the benefits of the DEU is the most effective way to promote the DEU. This book represents an undertaking by all contributors to ensure the DEU's ongoing evolution, uptake and sustainability.

Where to Next for DEUs?

The DEU strategy works. It has been consolidated across different levels of university and organisation leadership and endorsed as a sustainable solution to the global issue of having to find clinical learning placements for increasing numbers of nursing students. The agility of the DEU strategy is self-evident. You can implement DEUs differently in different settings or contexts, within the same university or health-care organisation or across different universities and health-care organisations. The DEU's ability to accommodate students across year levels at the same time, encouraging and developing peer teaching and learning as an additional skill, with a focus on communication and support, adds to its plausibility as a model for interprofessional education.

The DEU, originally conceived as a flexible strategy for more effective clinical learning and more efficient administration in the cross-cultural context of collaborative university teaching and learning and health service clinical teaching and learning, requires further crafting to meet different context-specific needs with different personnel and different organisations. Further expansion is anticipated in the area of interprofessional DEUs, which will expand the clinical knowledge of all students and clinical and academic staff about how to work in an interprofessional care team, how to value interprofessional information and share it and how to provide more informed care for patients.

Dedicated Education Units also have the potential for greater academic engagement with curriculum and research, engagement borne out of the relationships developed within the units as exemplified by nurse researcher Ann Harrington in Story 11, Chap. 10 (this volume). Engagement in pedagogical and clinical research is a strategy for sustaining the DEU. This engagement will create stronger partnerships between universities and health-care organisations through students and academics working with clinical staff and organisation management on joint research projects within the clinical setting. This expanded collaboration will develop the evidence-based research that is currently missing from the partnership equation. DEUs can become a resource to support clinical research, a frame of reference for research with students, academics and clinicians that will benefit the health-care organisations, their patients/clients, the students, the clinical staff, the academics and the universities. However, this will not happen without committed leaders because, as Mulready-Shick and Flanagan have identified (2012), 'leadership is key to creating and sustaining partnerships such as DEUs'.

Finally, there is a need to develop a new evaluation tool to guide the DEU process in the future and to enhance its credibility among those trying to understand the concept or sceptical about how it works. Further evaluation and dissemination of the findings across all health sciences and other human services disciplines who currently work in the same clinical spaces can open the door to developing interprofessional DEUs. Such development would require consideration of each profession's curriculum, planning and assessment approaches (Henderson and Alexander 2011). However, the way the DEU works, with students and clinical and academic staff working together as a team, provides the ideal environment for expansion to interprofessional teamwork. It is time to get the health and human service professions together to trial and evaluate interprofessional DEUs.

References

Cooper, L., Orrell, J., & Bowden, M. (2010). *Work integrated learning: A guide to effective practice*. London: Routledge.

Flash, P., Froehlich, J., Helgeson, S., Jensen, J. T., & Biotti, J. S. (2006). *Identifying key attributes of an effective transformational change model at the University of Minnesota*. Minneapolis: University of Minnesota: 2005–2006 President's Emerging Leader Team. http://www1.umn.edu/ohr/prod/groups/ohr/@pub/@ohr/documents/asset/ohr_65741.pdf. Accessed 20 Oct 2010.

Henderson, A., & Alexander, H. (2011). Maximising the integration of medical and nursing students in clinical learning environments: An Australian perspective. In S. Billett & A. Henderson (Eds.), *Developing learning professionals: Integrating experiences in university and practice settings* (pp. 131–148). Dordrecht: Springer.

Mulready-Shick, J., & Flanagan, K. (2012). *Project PDQ–Partnering for DEU development and quality*. http://www.evaluatinginnovationsinnursing.org/our-grantees/massachusetts/ Accessed 27 Feb 2013.

Sims, D. (2008). *Destination DEU. Getting started: A New Zealand experience*. PowerPoint presentation to National Nurse Education Conference, Sydney, Australia.

Glossary

The terminology used in this book reflects the contributions from authors in different parts of the world. The words 'academic', 'faculty' and 'teacher', for example, all refer to lecturers/teachers in universities. The terms clinician and clinical staff are used interchangeably throughout the book. Terminology used to describe the roles specific to different Dedicated Education Units (DEUs) also varies. This glossary provides a guide to the different terms used for the same, similar and different roles within DEUs in different locations. It has four sections: 'Clinical Lecturer' roles (university staff); 'Clinical Educator' roles (clinical staff/clinicians); 'Coordinator' roles (university administration); and brief descriptions of other roles and specific clinical learning/teaching models.

Term	Acronym
Clinical Lecturer roles	
Academic Liaison Nurse: a permanent clinical lecturer at the university who provides consistent support to students and clinicians	ALN
Clinical Lecturer/Clinical Facilitator: academic staff who visit the clinical learning setting intermittently to provide curriculum integration and monitor the student's progress with the student and their preceptor; may also undertake research projects in the clinical setting	
Clinical Liaison Nurse/Dedicated Liaison Nurse/Liaison Nurse: an experienced Registered Nurse (RN) selected from the practice area who takes on extra responsibilities, including overseeing clinical learning in the DEU and liaising between staff, students and academics/faculty (particularly the ALN); the liaison between the unit and the university	CLN/DLN/LN
Clinical Scholar: an expert clinical nurse who meets the requirements for providing clinical education for nursing students, is a permanent member of clinical nursing staff on a medical unit and acts as a preceptor to new graduate Registered Nurses (RNs) and as a coach to staff preceptors	CS
Lead Teacher: academic staff in charge of both lecture and clinical components of a clinical course; responsible for assigning grades	

(continued)

K. Edgecombe and M. Bowden (eds.), *Clinical Learning and Teaching Innovations in Nursing*, Innovation and Change in Professional Education 10,
DOI 10.1007/978-94-007-7232-8,

(continued)

Term	Acronym
Primary Tutor: a Registered Nurse (RN) who has overall responsibility for conducting the students' clinical studies	
Principal Academic (PA): an academic lecturer in clinical (nursing school faculty member) who visits the clinical setting prior to student placement to facilitate clinical staff preparation for working with the students and thereafter visits the clinical setting regularly throughout each semester; communicates and liaises with students, the LN and the CNC, and utilises their ongoing expertise to facilitate students' learning	PA
Secondary Tutor: a Registered Nurse (RN) who guides the students in concrete care and learning situations or a certified nursing assistant who guides students during fundamental care procedures	
Clinical Educator roles	
Clinical Instructor: staff nurse who wants to teach	CI
Clinical Staff/Clinicians: Registered Nurses (RNs), Enrolled Nurses (ENs) and Assistants in Nursing (AIN) recognised as clinician educators for students, responsible for facilitating students' learning in collaboration with the Principal Academic (PA) and CLN/DLN/LN	
Registered Nurse: college or university qualified nurse licensed by a nursing registration body to undertake all facets of nursing in accordance with the body's regulations	RN
Enrolled Nurse: Diploma qualified nurse working under supervision of an RN to provide nursing care	EN
Assistants in Nursing: certificated nurses (not RNs) providing support to the nursing teams in clinical settings under supervision of RNs	AIN
Coordinator roles	
Clinical Faculty Coordinator: nursing faculty from the university who plans students' experience and informs Clinical Instructors (CI) what is covered in university classes each week	CFC
Clinical Placement Coordinator: academic/faculty in the university responsible for negotiating clinical placements and ensuring placements are congruent with curriculum requirements	CPC
Other terminology	
Block placement: students placed in clinical setting for a short, concentrated block of time, overseen by clinical facilitators	
Capacity building: preparation/orientation for the DEU for academic and clinical staff, plus ongoing professional development pertinent to academic and clinical staff roles and responsibilities in the DEU environment	
Cluster model: block placement with one clinical facilitator working with a group of students and two RNs	
Community of practice: a community of people involved in mutual engagement (a network of multiple relationships between members of the community), having a shared repertoire ('routines, words, tools, ways of doing things, stories, gestures, symbols, genres, actions or concepts that the community has produced or adopted in the course of its existence') (Wenger 1998: 83) and collectively negotiating day-to-day practice (joint enterprise)	

(continued)

(continued)

Term	Acronym
Director of Nursing: An RN who supervises a whole nursing department	DON
Lifeworld perspective: a fundamental approach to learning in which the learner's world of experiences (i.e. their lifeworld) is the starting point for all learning support	
Magnet Hospital: a hospital that has been awarded recognition by the American Nurses Credentialing Center as a hospital that demonstrates excellence in nursing care	
Peer learning: learning with and from peers	
Preceptor/mentor: an experienced RN who provides one-on-one support for nursing students	
Preceptorship model: one student allocated to one preceptor (RN)	

Reference

Wenger, E. (1998). *Communities of practice: Learning, meaning and identity*. Cambridge: Cambridge University Press.

MIX
Papier aus verantwortungsvollen Quellen
Paper from responsible sources
FSC® C105338

If you have any concerns about our products,
you can contact us on
ProductSafety@springernature.com

In case Publisher is established outside the EU,
the EU authorized representative is:
Springer Nature Customer Service Center GmbH
Europaplatz 3, 69115 Heidelberg, Germany

Printed by Libri Plureos GmbH
in Hamburg, Germany